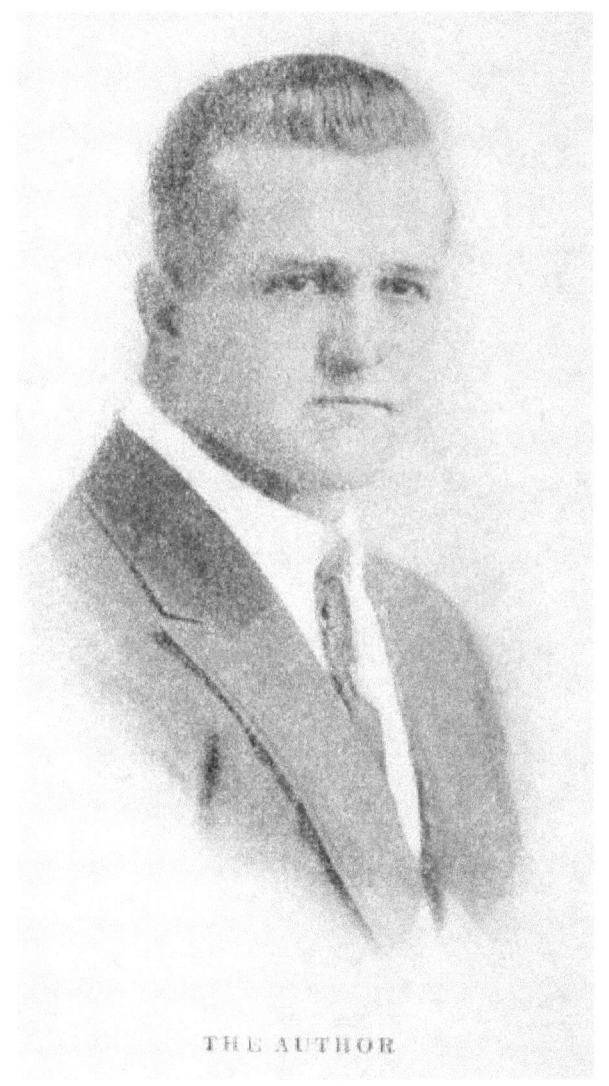

THE AUTHOR

ENDURANCE
(ORIGINAL VERSION, RESTORED)

By
EARLE LIEDERMAN

Originally Published in 1926

PUBLISHED BY O'Faolain Patriot LLC, Copyright 2011
info@PhysicalCultureBooks.com
Published in the United States of America

ISBN-13: 978-1466433878

ISBN-10: 1466433876

To Order More Copies Visit: Physical Culture Books.com

TABLEOFCONTENTS

INTRODUCTION

It is hard, sometimes, when one is busy, to leave mail unanswered and close up the desk and leave the city for a week or two, but that is just what I did. I packed my grip and departed one cold December day for the Southland.

I have a cozy little spot on the sands of Florida to where I have journeyed so many times to be alone with my thoughts and to write. Most of the books I have written were jotted down under the semi-tropical sun; and as I have had so many hundreds of requests from the readers of my athletic library for a book on endurance, I decided the time was ripe to take about twenty pencils and a ream of paper and get on the job to satisfy the thirst of my many friends and readers who want to learn my ideas and views on this subject.

While sitting on the sands, wondering how to begin this book, I noticed coming towards me, about one hundred feet away, a veritable giant. My eyes were held steady by his enormous breadth and massive chest. I doubt whether I have ever seen before such a chest, so barrel-like in dimensions. I watched every step he took. I did not notice his Herculean legs until he drew near me. Much to my surprise, who should it be but Henry Elionsky, who is without a doubt the most spectacular endurance swimmer the world ever produced. I had met him once before, a great many years ago, and had almost forgotten about him. That is why I did not recognize his gigantic physique until his features became distinguishable. Then, too, his mustache hindered my recognition.

I surely was glad to see him. Here I was about to begin writing on endurance; and what could be more fitting than to meet a man who, without a doubt, has the greatest endurance of any swimmer on earth? It seemed too good to be true. After the usual reminiscences, Mr. Elionsky gave me quite a lot of valuable information regarding endurance.

First of all, he claimed that the motive or goal was the first requisite towards prolonging motion. To use his own words:

"If, when swimming, you have no object or goal in view you will never swim as far as your will power tells you to. Although my muscles never become tired, still in order to swim twenty-five or thirty miles I naturally would have to set my destination.

"One essential thing about endurance is that the swimmer must learn the art of relaxation. Unless every part of the body is relaxed and you know the proper method of breathing, you never will become an endurance swimmer.

"I remember the time I swam from New York to Sandy Hook, N. J., a distance of about twenty-six miles, with my hands and feet tied and at the same time towing a rowboat containing a dozen men. There was a strong wind blowing against me and, although I gauged the tides, nevertheless the tide turned after I was in the water for eight hours. If on this occasion I had not absolutely relaxed every part of my body; if there had been one single muscle under tension, I would never have been able to successfully accomplish this unprecedented feat; or if I had on one single occasion gotten water in my nasal or air passage of my mouth, it would have so greatly interfered with my breathing that I would have been compelled to give up shortly after. I was compelled to adopt perfect breathing in the water.

"I am thinking seriously of making the attempt to swim the English Channel with my hands and feet shackled. I am positive I can do it, and although I have never been across the ocean to try out the channel, still I know for a positive fact that as long as I practice the art of proper breathing and as long as my muscles are in a state of complete relaxation, I can successfully swim any distance within reason. Again, of course, the motive or the goal must be continually in my mind. If I simply took a swim, just for the sport of it, the chances are I would not swim more than two or three miles before I would feel as though I had had enough. But, realizing that I have a great distance to make, I must concentrate upon my destination.

"As an example, to show you what a valuable asset perfect breathing is to the swimmer, let me tell you of an incident that happened once while swimming Hell Gate Rapids. Hell Gate, as you know, connects the East River with Long Island Sound, and is filled with whirlpools and rocks. On this particular day I was to perform a freak swim, in which two men were strapped tightly to me, one on each side. I also had my hands and feet firmly tied. I was to swim the Hell Gate waters in this manner and, of course, for safety I had a couple of boats continually alongside of me.

"After about fifteen minutes in the water we struck a whirlpool. It dragged my feet down and thereby caused the weight of my human baggage to push me below the surface. I understand one of the men called out while my head was under water 'is everything all right?', but naturally I never heard him, and all I could do, when I struggled to the surface, was to look appealingly at the men in the accompanying boat. They, seeing my look, quickly pulled us out of the water.

"If we had not struck the little whirlpool, which caused this commotion, I would have as successfully swum these rapids as I have done on numerous other occasions. But being forced under the water by the combined weight of the two men strapped to me interfered so greatly with my breathing that it would have made it exceedingly difficult to continue. Had my hands been free, of course, it would have been easy."

This indicates quite clearly what such a great man as Elionsky thinks of relaxation, breathing, and having an object or goal in view. Personally, I really think that swimming calls for more endurance than any other sport, because not only must the destination be continually in the mind, but one must battle with the waves and at the same time breathe rhythmically. No matter how strenuous a sport one undertakes on land, whether it be boxing, wrestling, tennis, running, or the like, there is always air at the command of the lungs; but in swimming, where the face is so much under water and the head must be turned to get the air, it is much more difficult to secure the necessary oxygen.

Probably an endurance swimmer would make a very poor Marathon runner and an impossible boxer or wrestler, just as the world's champion boxer or wrestler would, ninetynine times out of a hundred, make an impossible endurance swimmer, as every athlete has a specialty in some line or other. But everyone can learn and practice the rudiments of the different sports or pastimes and become better at any of them than the average. Some of our lightweight fighters, who can box twenty or more rounds at top speed, and some of our heavyweight wrestlers, who can keep up the pace hour after hour, perhaps could swim several miles should they go in for endurance swimming; but they would fall far short of the distances covered by Elionsky or any other endurance swimmer.

And that reminds me that, after I left Mr. Elionsky, I had not gone a hundred yards before I met Budd Goodwin, the former world's champion endurance swimmer. Mr. Goodwin has won more cups and gold medals than any other living athlete; they number into the thousands; and he still holds one record that never has been duplicated. Mr. Goodwin's favorite pastime was swimming a distance of thirteen miles from New York to Coney Island, and his remarkable speed, combined with his endurance, has made him one of the greatest swimmers of all times.

I have asked Mr. Goodwin on one or two occasions what he thinks about when swimming mile after mile. His answer always has been the same: "I must not give up; I must reach my goal." Here again is indication that a destination or goal plays an important part in a swimmer's career. Of course, no matter what the goal may be, no swimmer would make it if he did not absolutely relax and understand perfect form in breathing. By the way, never in all my life have I seen such remarkable breathing as that practiced by Budd Goodwin. To watch him swim is a treat. It seems that his face is continually in the water and that he never takes a breath; but his great speed forms a little pocket under his nose, as he turns his head slightly sideways, and it is in this pocket that he secures his air. I doubt whether anyone else is as proficient in the art of breathing while swimming as is Budd Goodwin.

In one of my other books, Secrets of Strength, I asked the question, "What is endurance but continued strength?" If one were to have the pleasure of beholding either Mr. Elionsky or Mr. Goodwin in person, he would see before him a powerful man of gigantic physique; and, although Mr. Elionsky's chest is considerably greater than Mr. Goodwin's (measuring, I believe, fifty-eight inches normal), still Mr. Goodwin has such a massive lung space that his depth and breadth of chest would look well on a two hundred and fifty pound wrestler, yet he weighs but two hundred pounds.

Thus it will be appreciated that the first requisite for the student in acquiring endurance is to learn the art of relaxation and to have a destination in mind, whether it be in swimming, skating, boxing, wrestling, or any other form of athletic sport. While the art of proper breathing is very essential in swimming, it forms perhaps a somewhat lesser part in other pastimes.

An example of complete relaxation can be illustrated as follows: hold your arm sideways at the height of your shoulder and have someone place his hands under your wrist and forearm, letting the entire weight of your arm rest on his hands; then have him, without warning, quickly pull his hands away. If your arm quickly drops downward and hits against your side, that arm is in a state of relaxation. But if it lowers slowly or does not reach the side, your deltoid or shoulder muscle has been slightly tensed.

If you can learn to relax each and every muscle of your body and just flop, so to speak, it will help you a good deal in training for any kind of endurance. About the only place one can completely relax is in the water; for while a bed may be soft, still the mattress or springs will cause some minor part of your body to be in a slight tension. In the water, however—it being buoyant—you can find absolute relaxation after you have mastered this art.

The reader must pardon me if I seem to ramble too deeply into the subject in this introduction; but as this book is being written as I go along, naturally I am anxious to jot down the various thoughts and ideas as they loom before me. I must not be blamed for my enthusiasm nor for having written the highlights of my fortunate meeting with two such interesting men as Elionsky and Goodwin. There I sat with the warm sun glaring down upon me, biting the top of my pencil and wondering how to begin, when these living inspirations of endurance suddenly seemed to come to me from nowhere. Now that I have quoted them and the literary error has been committed and I am once again alone with my thoughts, I hope you who read this will be as interested in what I shall write as I shall be in writing the following chapters for you.

ENDURANCE

I

EVERY man should be able to save his own life. He should be able to swim far enough, run fast and long enough to save his life in case of emergency and necessity. He also should be able to chin himself a reasonable number of times, as well as to dip a number of times, and he should be able to jump a reasonable height and distance.

If he is of the fat, porpoise type, naturally he cannot do all, if any, of these things; and he has nobody to blame but himself, and his way of living that has brought his body into its condition of obesity.

Suppose—and it has happened many times—there should be a fire at sea or on lake or river; should one be half a mile or more from the shore, he would be mighty thankful to realize, were he compelled to jump for his life from the fire, that he could swim that distance and reach the short in safety.

Suppose one were in a burning building and he had to lower himself hand under hand down a rope or down an improvised rope of bedclothing tied together to reach the ground in safety; he again would be thankful a thousand times that he possessed the strength and endurance in his arms and coordinate muscles that would enable him to save himself. Such things never may happen, and let us hope they do not; but what has happened always is possible to occur again—and, in fact, always is happening to some one.

While I was in the lobby of a Southern hotel one winter evening, two men came in with a large rattlesnake hanging on a pole. These two men had been out that day hunting rabbits and other small game, and one of the men in stepping over a small stone fence surrounding a farm suddenly beheld this rattlesnake coiled up not three feet from him, with tail swishing and ready to spring. The reader may know that a rattlesnake always can spring its own length. The man, who had stepped with one leg over the wall, had sufficient presence of mind to realize that if he moved a muscle the snake would spring. Therefore, he stood motionless, straddling this wall, one leg about three feet from the snake and the other leg in the grass on the other side of the stones. After remaining motionless for what he said seemed a long time, he finally nerved himself and with every ounce of strength he possessed in his legs he jumped with both feet sideways so that he cleared the wall and rolled on the ground on the other side of the stones, miraculously escaping the lunge of the rattler. As he sprang to his feet his partner quickly came to his assistance and killed the snake, which had plunged over the two-foot wall, missing the other man's leg by but a few inches.

Such incidents in the life of men seem incredible—in the realm of fiction; but it nevertheless is a true story. And, again, what has happened once may be repeated. If this man had not possessed the strong quality of muscle in his legs, developed by his constant cross-country walking (for he hunted regularly), he would not have had the ability nor the confidence to spring suddenly, as he did, to escape the poisonous bite of the reptile.

In my younger days I had to run quite a distance over the fields, at top speed, to escape the charge of a mad bull. At the end of the fields was the common farm fence; you know the kind—cross bars and jagged ends sticking up here and there. I think no one ever hurdled or vaulted with greater speed than I did on that occasion. Another rare incident—yet it happened to me; and if I had not been able to run with speed and jump or vault over the old farm fence with such quickness, there might be a different story to tell. This is another example proving the value of endurance and well trained muscles.

Last year, while on the beach at Atlantic City, N. J., I was introduced to a robust fellow whose arm was in a sling. Naturally I asked him what had happened. He told me that the day before there was a railroad wreck, of which I had heard, not far from Atlantic City. The train was speeding at the rate of about sixty miles an hour when the rails spread, and as the train jumped the track all the coaches overturned. This fellow by chance happened to be roaming in the meadows within a hundred yards of the tracks and, therefore, saw the whole catastrophe. It is hard to relate twice-told tales accurately, but he told me how he ran quickly toward the wreck as he heard the uncanny screams of the injured passengers. Time after time he climbed over a capsized car, entered the broken windows and helped the injured out of safety. Still the moans kept up. He told me his legs and arms were shaking from the fatigue of lifting and carrying the people away from the wreck; he was ready to drop. Yet he carried on, and it was in the attempt to rescue a screaming woman, who was pinned underneath one of the cars which had toppled over, that he received his injury. This car rested upon one of the trucks or set of wheels. While under this truck, which evidently was on meager balance, his arm was smashed by the collapse of the wreckage. This is an instance well illustrating the value of endurance. Think how many more lives might have been lost had this fellow not possessed the physical power to continue. If endurance may not prove useful in saving your own life, it may prove exceedingly valuable in saving the lives of others.

A man does not necessarily need to be a strong man or even a muscular athlete in order to possess endurance qualities necessary to save his own life. Neither does one need youth, as counted in years; for even in middle life a reasonable amount of endurance can be gotten by anyone who really wants it. But if the individual contents himself with living a life of ease and inactivity, drinking, smoking, over-indulging in food, and giving way to feelings or emotions, he must not expect anything but shortness of breath, unnecessary flesh, unresponsive nerves and muscles, and a sluggish mind.

I do not believe in everyone striving to be a long distance swimmer, a long distance runner, or any other kind of endurance athlete. The performance of such work necessary to acquire great endurance in all these things would, especially in later years, endanger the heart. But he should be able to swim at least half a mile or more; he should be able to run at top speed two hundred yards or more; he should be able to jump over obstacles higher than his waist; and he should be in condition to pull his body upward by the strength of his arms, until his chin touches his hands, at least fifteen to twenty times; and as for pushing ability, he should be able to dip between parallel bars or between two chairs at least twenty-five times or more. If he can accomplish these things he need have no fear concerning the safety of his life should he be forced into an emergency from which he alone may be able to save himself.

I shall not devote any space to methods of acquiring a well-proportioned and strong body, for in my book Muscle Building I have gone into this matter in detail. From this brief chapter concerning the saving of your own life and the possession of sufficient strength, endurance, coordination and responsiveness of muscles to make it possible for one to save his life, I think the reader will be more interested in learning how to acquire this reasonable amount of endurance and other qualities, which may prove essential at some time during his lifetime.

II

WHILE it is true that I am an advocate of muscle building and strength work, perhaps it is because I am still living the best years of my life, and my enthusiasm is just as keen now as it was twenty-five years ago. But I am as positive as I am of my writing this that the time will come, as my years increase, when my desire to continue my strenuous physical activities will lessen; and I know when that time comes my greatest enthusiasm in regard to the physical will be toward retaining my robust health. Strength and muscles for the sake of these alone no longer will be of interest. This is simply a law of human nature. What does a man of sixty care about competitive strength or bulging muscles? His main goal in life should be the maintenance or development of robust health and vitality.

Let the reader not misunderstand me and think that this book is a book for the older man. It is not. It is written for the benefit of all ages. But as the healthy, enthusiastic youth naturally possesses the seemingly tireless energy, I feel as though the word "endurance" will be of more interest to the one who used to be "good" and who has slipped backward—the man of middle life who recalls with longing thoughts the vigorous youth and young man that he used to be. How many times do the words enter your mind, "I used to be able to do that when I was younger," etc. I always dislike to hear anyone say these things, for, if he is not boasting, he is acknowledging that he has led such a life of physical inactivity or self-indulgence as to become— if not really a "has been," a "never was." There really is no excuse for anyone to deteriorate physically quicker than nature intended, and nature surely meant the man of forty to be in his prime of life. But how many are, at this age? Most of them are "has beens," and look much older than their years. The man of sixty or sixty-five should be in just as good health and have practically as much vitality as he had when he was thirty. Suppose a few gray hairs do appear, or a couple of lines gather on the face; what should they matter as long as he feels and acts physically like a youth of twenty-five?

Endurance work is the only exercising that the aged man, the man with the weak heart, the consumptive, or even the beginner, should indulge in, and in these cases it must be of a gentle variety and not severe enough to cause fatigue. For the man with the weak heart or the man past middle life the endurance work must be so gentle as to prevent any strain whatsoever. It should be done slowly enough and with enough pause between each two movements to give the organs and muscles a chance to recuperate.

An example of this can be gotten from walking. Put a man with a weak heart walking up a hill or a grade and the work, instead of being an exercise of simple endurance form, becomes an exercise of fatigue; whereas, even in such a condition, walking on level ground may be prolonged hour after hour without fatigue. Progression in the exercise can be made by increasing the rapidity of the steps, but this should be done very systematically and, preferably, under careful guidance.

The best example of endurance is shown by the heart. It begins work several months before birth and ceases only with death; and the only reason it is capable of such continuous contractions is because the cardiac or heart muscle rests after each heart beat, thereby recuperating sufficiently to continue beating. If the heart is overexerted through undue physical activity that greatly quickens its action or beats, the cardiac muscle cannot recuperate quickly enough and the heart becomes overtaxed.

The same thing applies to all the other muscles of the body. When exercises are indulged in which produce rapid physical fatigue, the work is strength-increasing and muscle-building; but a complete relaxation and rest must follow such a period of strenuous exercise in order to give the muscles a chance to recuperate. Otherwise the tissues will be torn down more quickly than they can be replenished and the only progress will be backward, in development, strength and energy.

No better illustration of this can be had than that of a professional circus strong man (I do not recall his name) who years ago possessed such stubborn determination regarding his exercising that it became an obsession with him. Not only was he compelled to perform numerous exhibitions in the sideshow where he worked, but his determination to add more and more muscle to his frame stimulated him to exercise for long periods at a time, several times a day. This he kept up month after month and year after year. But instead of his muscles growing larger and larger, they became smaller and smaller, until he died, in the prime of life. Just before his untimely death he was so nervous and thin from his self-destructive practice that he not only proved useless as an exhibitor but he developed a pale, emaciated appearance. This man positively killed himself by overwork, by prolonging his exercises beyond the time when he should have stopped; and instead of relaxing and resting and giving his muscles a chance to grow, he wore himself out.

I recall another case, that of a young man I met by chance many years ago, who was deeply interested in feats of strength and physical development in general. His one desire seemed to be to get muscularly strong. Judging by his thin, nervous appearance that there was a drain upon his vitality, I inquired into his methods of training, and learned that he exercised every day for two or three hours at a time. I told him to cut down on his training and not to exercise more than one-half hour each day, and if he found that he did not put on more weight in a short time and if his muscles did not increase in size and his strength improve, he should exercise for one-half hour every other day. It gave me as much pleasure then to advise this young fellow as it does today to guide my enthusiastic pupils. This young man soon passed out of my mind, and it was only recently that I again, by chance, met him in another city which I was visiting. He was still thin, appearing to be not one pound heavier than when I had seen him several years ago. I asked him if he still continued exercising, and if he were as interested in physical development now as he used to be. He told me he was more enthusiastic than ever and that he exercised faithfully. He still persisted with his daily training for an hour or two at a time. The only thing I could do was to repeat my advice, but I felt that it merely went in one ear and out the other. Think of all the energy this fellow has wasted year after year, exercising for less than nothing! He is getting no stronger and no heavier, neither are his muscles increasing in size or contour; he is simply burning up tissues and wasting his energy as quickly as, if not quicker, than they can be restored.

In the case of this young man and in that of the circus performer mentioned previously, the exercising they did must be termed endurance work, and no human being can keep up strenuous, heavy endurance exercise, working hour after hour, without exhaustion of physical and nervous energies. These cases prove that endurance exercises prolonged by will power beyond the point of fatigue and repeated too often, will do more injury than good to the body.

I have emphasized the value of walking as an endurance movement. Rowing is another form of exercise that should be indulged in by those whose hearts are weak or whose years forbid heavier exertions. Whether this rowing is done on calm water or on a rowing machine, the movements can be done slowly enough and in such a mechanical way that the weakest individual can keep it up for a long period of time, usually with only beneficial results. If, on the other hand, the pace is quickened the work enters the class of muscle-building and strength-producing exercises and would prove too violent for a weak heart.

Now the question arises, when is exercise endurance work and when is it muscle-building work? What is endurance work for one may prove muscle-building work for another, and vice versa. This all depends upon the individual's strength. If a healthy young man were to go out rowing and row mechanically and slowly, with just enough pause between each two strokes to permit recuperation, he could continue hour after hour and perhaps all day; and, if he has never done this work before, the only unpleasant results arising from such a lengthy row would be a callous or two on his hands and perhaps a few sore muscles the next day. Therefore, it would seem useless and a waste of energy for any strong, healthy young man to indulge in such a light pastime unless it were done merely for pleasure.

On the other hand, should the individual have a weak heart or should he be in the declining years of life, such a long row would prove too fatiguing and would, without a doubt, overtax his heart and energies. Such an individual naturally should begin such endurance work, in the initial attempt, only for very brief periods of time. A fifteenminute row should be sufficient for the first time, and should never under any circumstances be done in rough water, or against any great resistance if performed on the rowing machine. He will find it an easy matter to row for thirty minutes or even one hour after a sufficient time of mild preparation, providing, of course, sufficient brief pause is put in between strokes for recuperative purposes.

Walking should be progressed in the same manner— first a stroll, and at some later time the pace quickened according to the strength of the individual. That is one reason why golf is an ideal recreation for the older man, although it is not an old man's game by any means. The links are full of youths and most of the top-notchers in this game are comparatively young men.

Have you ever watched day laborers digging in the streets or working on railroad tracks? If you have you may have wondered how they could keep that work up all day long, day after day—that is if you have ever tried similar work yourself. The next time you observe a day laborer note how slowly he works. There is no haste in picking up things or moving, though should the gang foreman be around there perhaps may be more effort put forth than at other times; but as soon as the foreman leaves you will find the laborers straightening up and relaxing, even though it be for but a moment or two at a time. If it were not for this relaxation at every opportunity, and the slowness with which they work while actually "on the job," pausing between actions, they would not be able to continue their labor. Should you wish to experiment in this line yourself, just go out and shovel snow some winter day, and you will find that you cannot keep it up very long if you use the shovel with enthusiasm.

I remember that one year when returning from Europe there was a shipping strike in Sweden. The boat had to sail on time and the crew was composed mostly of young college students who volunteered to work on the boat for their passage to America. I had the good fortune to become acquainted with the staff captain, who was very hospitable in showing me around the ship. After we were a few days out we encountered very heavy seas, caused by a hurricane which had been blowing all night. The boat was pitching and tossing and the waves washed over the bow on many occasions. Fortunately I possess a stomach not easily disturbed and I never get seasick; so I gladly accepted the staff captain's invitation to visit the engine room, as he previously had informed me that owing to the storm there was more work than ever to be performed in the engine room and one after another these young students were fainting from the heat. So down we went, deck below deck, until the air became hot and stuffy. There I saw these young fellows, some stripped to the waist, working frantically without pause, it seemed. I marvelled at their endurance, and it was no wonder to me that they became exhausted and dropped from the exertion and the heat. Yet the work had to go on. The engines had to be fired. It was difficult to stand, owing to the rolling of the boat, which caused additional work for the muscles of the laborers in order to maintain body balance. This was just another illustration proving to me that relaxation is necessary, and a pause must be placed between movements. Otherwise, the limit of endurance quickly will be reached and the body will collapse.

Not so many years ago Marathon races were the craze in New York City. Around and around the track of the old Madison Square Garden these runners would go, one after the other; and it was only the goal they had in mind and the indomitable will power they had that propelled their legs even after their bodily inclinations said "stop." The result was that at the finish all would be at a point of exhaustion, and many would collapse.

Now another question arises: How much can the human body endure and with safety? It is known that a man can outrun in endurance a horse, for it has been done. We can go without sleep day after day; we can go without food or drink for an almost unbelievable time. But it is interesting to note the reaction in each instance. In the matter of exercise, if the reaction after endurance work is one of severe fatigue, it proves that the movements have been carried on for too long a time. Of course, when endurance work is done as in case of necessity or in case of competition, fatigue must be expected, and such physical exertion should not be classed as exercise.

I think I am safe in classifying as endurance work any movement that can be performed with the arms over one hundred repetitions; and yet here is another example of strength work almost entering the endurance classification. In the rear part of my office I have a number of heavy barbells. I keep these on hand to test the strength of my pupils when they visit me from time to time. One day one of my star pupils asked me to show him certain methods of performing a difficult lift. While there I jokingly told I would hold with him a contest in lifting. I picked up a bar-bell which weighed either one hundred pounds or one hundred and twenty pounds. (I do not recall at the present writing which weight.) I remember lifting it over my head, with two hands, about fifty or sixty times. Then I asked him to see how many times he could perform this lift. I thought I would prove to be the winner, for at about his forty-fifth count I remember how much his back started to bend and with what difficulty he was pressing it overhead; but at the seventy-fifth count he was continuing, with the same difficulty and the same arch in his back. I marveled at the wonderful endurance his muscles possessed, and yet he was lifting a bar-bell—strength work.

This, again, shows that what is strength work for one is endurance work for another; and although seventy-five repetitions or more cannot bring the exercise strictly under the endurance class, it at least shows continued strength. And, in the final analysis, continued strength is very closely related to endurance; they seem to go hand in hand. To lift with one hand a fifty-pound dumbbell from the floor to arm's length overhead and lower again would prove quite a difficult feat of strength for a weak chap. Yet I have seen this same young man mentioned above perform this lift three hundred and fifty times without stopping.

So many times I give my students the common push-up exercise to be performed on the floor. Undoubtedly you are familiar with this movement, which consists of lying flat on the abdomen and, while keeping the body rigid, pushing up with the arms and lowering until tired. For beginners this movement is muscle-building work, but after a few months it ceases to be valuable as progressive exercising and turns into an endurance movement. I, myself, have performed this movement over one hundred and fifty times without stopping, and I know of other strong men who have accomplished this.

To lie flat on the back, with the hands placed behind the head, and then come to a sitting posture until the elbows touch the knees may prove quite an effort to one who never has done it before; yet this same movement has been done over two thousand and seven hundred times without stopping.

Some people have difficulty even in bending their knees without their joints cracking. To one who never has squatted, ten or fifteen squats would make the muscles of the thighs exceedingly lame the next day. I recall one stout woman attempting to do the squat exercise or sitting on her heels, but after lowering the body she was unable to rise again by the strength of her thigh muscles. Yet this same movement has been done over three thousand times without stopping.

How winded and exhausted the average man becomes after running one block to catch his train in the morning! And yet Paavo Nurmi will run mile after mile and at the finish appear comparatively fresh, in wind, strength and energy.

Have you ever watched the efforts of a beginner learning to swim? After twenty or thirty feet he must come out of the water, before exhaustion overtakes him. And yet Henry Elionsky, while forced to abandon an attempt to swim one hundred miles, did swim over thirty miles, in spite of the tide and rough sea that forced him to discontinue.

I relate these instances merely to show you that what is strength work for one is endurance work for another; so, therefore, what is endurance but continued strength?

III

ENDURANCE work cannot be performed rapidly. It must be done slowly, but without thought of count. So many devotees to physical exercise set a certain number of counts as their goal. This is all well and good for setting-up exercises; but when the mind is continually concentrating upon figures some nervous energy is wasted, which could be utilized either in accomplishing results or for a useful purpose. Monotony soon becomes evident when counting, serving to detract from the interest of the work; also, counting is inclined to cause one to throw less energy into his muscles for beneficially greater contraction. Therefore, exercising simply to reach an allotted number of counts is not as beneficial as when a destination or physiological goal is the object.

It is much better, for example, to set your goal in walking, say, at one or two miles than to count your steps. If the student should be exercising with light dumbbells it is much better to continue until the muscles feel tired than simply to set out to do one hundred or two hundred lifts regardless of the consequences. The number of counts may be easy some days, but too much on other days. The object of performing endurance exercises is to do the work in the easiest way possible, with just enough pause between movements to give the tissues and the heart action a chance to recuperate. Without relaxation in endurance work the work becomes muscle-building and strength-building rather than endurance in nature.

I really believe the phlegmatic type of person possesses more power of endurance than the nervous type. The nervous individual consumes or wastes his energy not only in muscular effort but mental effort as well. If you tell a nervous person to quickly touch a button and turn on a light he will do it much quicker than his phlegmatic friend. There are exceptions to this rule, and in fact this may be only my personal opinion; but most of the endurance athletes I have met have been of the steady, easy-going, nonexcitable type.

This does not mean, at all, that one of nervous temperament cannot develop much endurance. While they are, as a rule, more fitted for rapid or speed work, and while they naturally "take to" this class of work in their physical activities and sports, yet they can develop an endurance for such work that is equal to that possessed by the phlegmatic athletes who generally take up slower activities. Since the nervous energy of the man of nervous temperament is inclined to burn out more quickly, though perhaps burning at "greater heat"—permitting more intense work while it endures—the work done by such a person to help develop endurance, should be done more slowly than is his natural inclination. Of course, there may be some fast work, and usually there should be a goodly proportion of such; but in heavier work and definite endurance there must be a "toning down," a slowing down, for best results.

Good lungs are essential for anyone who is desirous of accomplishing anything in the endurance. If there is shortness of breath, exhaustion will soon set in. Any of you who have attended amateur boxing exhibitions (I do not mean professional, for professional boxers usually are in good condition and have excellent wind) have noted the difference in the action in the various rounds. In the first round two amateur boxers will rush at each other like angry bulls. The second round is a little slower, and often one of the contestants slows up so appreciably that one can but wonder what has become of all his ferociousness. It is a matter of becoming winded through too violent exercise early in the fight.

I remember attending an amateur boxing show at the New York Athletic Club where there was a husky chap introduced as Sailor somebody. His body was superbly developed and he looked as if he could tear his opponent in two. When the bell sounded for the first round he tore in and showered blows upon his adversary so that after but a minute or so of fighting his opponent began to appear groggy from the onslaught. However, his more frail appearing opponent managed to weather the round. In the second round this husky boxer started with the same ferociousness, but before many seconds had elapsed he quite suddenly slowed down. Then came the other fellow's turn, and it wasn't long before the muscular marvel was lying outstretched upon the floor. He slowed up so noticeably that he was an easy mark for his opponent, who possessed better endurance qualities—and, incidentally, the necessary punch.

Do you suppose Harry Greb, the middleweight boxer, could continue at top speed round after round for fifteen or twenty rounds or more, if he did not relax his muscles absolutely in between encounters, blocks or punches, and if he did not possess a wonderful pair of lungs? I have seen Johnny Dundee, the former featherweight champion, for twenty rounds hit so fast and so often and jump around so constantly that it seemed incredible for a human being to keep up the pace. Anyone who has tried boxing will realize the value of good "wind." Both Greb and Dundee, of course, are exceptions in the boxing world, just as Elionsky, Goodwin, Nurmi, and others are exceptions in their own sports.

It is the exceptions that make the champions; but for the average competitor in any sport that requires endurance, whether it be boxing twenty rounds, swimming or running several miles, or what not, the start always should be moderate, and then this moderate pace should be kept up throughout the entire performance, or at least until second wind has developed. Suppose you were punching the bag; if you went at it top speed it would require a good deal of wind, as well as strength in the arms and shoulders, and you soon would find yourself tiring. In my opinion, this manner of bag-punching would be considered musclebuilding work. On the other hand, suppose you wished to punch the bag for an hour or two at a time. You would not attempt rapidity of movement; you would, naturally, take it easy, and the bag would not hit the platform as rapidly as it would ordinarily in swift work.

Our professional wrestlers, whom you often may have seen wrestle for an hour or two at a time, in most cases are given a certain allotted time in which to wrestle. If these athletes are required to wrestle for an hour in order to give the public an interesting exhibition, as well as its money's worth, you do not see them tear at each other like mad bulls. If you are a student or devotee of the game you would find evidence of plenty of relaxation, in spite of the fact that they appear continually to exert all their strength.

Yet it is remarkable how much the human body can endure. I know of chaps who go on continually dissipating and who apparently are strong and husky; but are they? I often wonder what interesting things one might behold if it were possible for one to see the inside of their bodies.

Perhaps you have heard the story about the frog who was boiled to death; but it may be new to some, so I relate it. In one of our leading universities some experimenters placed a bullfrog into a pan of cool water. This pan was then placed upon a heater and the temperature of the water was increased so slowly that it took over one hour for the water to come to the boiling point. During all this time the frog never moved. He was slowly boiled to death, yet gave no evidence of feeling the rising heat.

How many people are like that frog! They continue their dissipated way of living and are slowly decaying without knowing it. Perhaps you may use intoxicants; you may smoke considerably, keep late hours, eat anything you like for perhaps a long time, and think you are getting away with it. But you are not! Just remember that a chain is no stronger than its weakest link, and that some day the weak link is going to snap! When it does you may never know it any more than the thousands who suddenly drop dead each day, though you may be even less fortunate than these, for the breaking of that weak link may be the beginning of years of broken health, perhaps with much physical suffering.

IV

DIET has a very important effect upon one's endurance, strength and nervous energy. The one who does not look after his diet will find his powers of endurance sadly slackening. Plain, wholesome food should be eaten at all times, and care should be taken as to the quantities and mixtures of certain foods that go into one's stomach. I am not going to completely discuss diet within these pages, for in one of my other books, Here's Healthy the reader will find a complete table of food values, as well as complete advice on food, hygiene, and physiology.

I am a firm believer in fruit juices for the benefit of the stomach. Anyone who has experienced drinking orange juice has found that considerable energy is derived from such a drink. It has been proven that vegetarians and those who eat plenty of fruit have more energy and endurance than meat eaters. The proper diet will keep the bowels in condition, and if their elimination process is functioning properly one will have greater powers of endurance than one would have if one were troubled with constipation or gases in the intestines or other disturbances resulting from defective elimination or other digestive disorders. In a following chapter I will present a further discussion of diet.

I am a firm believer in daily exercise, and I put this belief into practice. In my years of experience with training I have found that the best period for exercising is in the afternoon; but one cannot always take that time for his exercise period. Being just as busy as anyone else, I am forced to give up this best period for my work and to take my exercise in the morning upon arising. It sometimes is not easy to jump out of bed and begin a strenuous twenty minutes or so of exercising; but I have formed the habit of jumping under a cold shower to wake me up, so to speak.

After this cold bath, which I take winter and summer, I feel so pepped up that it is a pleasure to go through my exercises. This shower acts as a natural stimulant; and although I recommend it to those who can endure it and react from it, I would not recommend it to those who have a weak heart, especially an organically diseased heart, or to whom it would prove too much of a shock to the nerves. Some milder form of natural stimulant, therefore, would be better; and I suggest rubbing the body vigorously with a coarse towel and getting the blood into circulation in this manner. As soon as the blood is in brisk circulation the muscles will feel more alive and more like undertaking an exercise drill.

Only the other day a fellow asked me what I thought of stimulants to awaken the body before exercising, referring to artificial stimulants. He asked me what I thought of the use of coffee to whip up the nerves to get more force into movements, in other words using coffee as a stimulant. He claimed that when he first wakes in the mornings he does not have as much force to do his movements as after he drinks a cup of coffee. About fifteen to thirty minutes after having the coffee he feels like exercising. He claimed that drinking coffee at night affected his nerves to such an extent that he could not sleep, and, naturally, he was interested in knowing what effect the morning cup would have upon the muscles. I told him the effect of coffee would be on the nervous system and not on the muscles. Of course, if you stimulate your nerves to react more strongly than ordinarily, the muscles will respond better for a short time; but how about the reaction? I told him he reminded me very much of the circus strong man, whom I have mentioned in a previous chapter, who thought he simply had to do a movement a certain number of times every day. With him it was a sort of disease; and in spite of the fact that his muscles grew tired he had to keep on with the exercise until he had done each of his particular movements a certain number of counts. Naturally, he was forced to use a nerve stimulant in order to create the activity; and instead of improving in size, his muscles grew smaller and smaller because of the gradual exhaustion of his reserve nervous energy.

While I agree that a cup of coffee will stimulate you and keep you awake and enable you to exercise better, there is always a reaction or after-effect. Some authorities claim that a stimulant, if not overdone, will not harmfully effect you, but if overdone it positively will create a detrimental after-effect. However, the extent of the reaction in two different people is not the same. For instance, in a book on diet it relates how experiments with coffee were made upon two people. One of them after drinking a cup of coffee needed a physician to bring him back to health. Therefore, it readily can be seen that the nervous constitution of the person has to be taken into consideration. If a muscle is forced by a stimulant it will grow smaller eventually, for you cannot disregard nature's laws.

Recently I asked a friend of mine how he warmed up in the morning—did he take a cold shower upon arising, did he eat breakfast first to get his body in condition to exercise an hour later, or did he massage himself with a towel as I have previously suggested? He stated that when he got up in the morning he did not feel like exercising; in fact, he found it hard to even get up. Therefore, he started doing situps in bed. After doing ten or twelve of these he was awakened enough to do his leg work, first in bed and then out. By this time he was fully awake and able to stay out of bed and continue with the heavier work.

It seemed to me to be another good suggestion. Most people find it easier to start exercising slowly and warm up the muscles before attempting the heavier work, and I believe the majority of physical trainers consider this the more satisfactory method. But I have found just the opposite to be easier. I prefer to perform a few heavy movements, for after these heavy movements my muscles seem to be in condition to do anything. This, of course, may be an effect of the cold bath which I take before any exercise. An argument against my method is that there is a danger of straining a ligament by beginning the exercising with heavy work. It all depends upon the amount of resistance you are to work against and the capability of your muscles. I would not recommend anyone to lift a heavy weight, for instance, which was all he could lift when in his best condition for such work. If you are capable of lifting overhead one hundred and fifty pounds with two hands you never should make this lift the first thing upon arising, but rather should limit it to at most one hundred pounds. In other words, two thirds of your capability should be sufficient if you prefer to begin your morning exercise period in such a manner.

One's feelings or desire for exercise and activity differs greatly on different occasions, and the physical culturist who has experience with exercising will know this only too well. You may take the best of care of yourself, retire at the same time every night, be careful of your diet, and yet on the following day you may not possess the energy and vitality that you experienced the day before. Atmospheric conditions play an important part in this fluctuation of bodily forces. When the weather is rainy or the humidity high, we do not feel as energetic as we do in more favorable weather conditions.

I admit that when one is continually striving to perfect some physical accomplishment it is provoking to receive set-backs for no apparent reason. I recall my own experience in hand-balancing. I have been doing the exercise of standing on my hands ever since I can remember, and am always sure of performing a handstand in all of its variations of press-ups, etc., under almost any condition; but it took me a long, long time to master the one-hand stand. Just when I thought I had it and felt confident I could perform it, I found on the next day that I was all out of balance; I could not for the life of me seem to perform it half as well as I did on the day previous.

This has happened on numerous occasions in the past, and, undoubtedly, was due to the condition of my stomach which in turn reflected upon my vision, and also from the lack of proper coordinative balance in my muscles for this extremely exacting sort of exercise. Should there be the least bit of fermentation in the stomach it is apt to interfere somewhat with the sight, and eyesight in a one-hand stand, in my estimation, plays an important part, as the eyes must be focussed on one spot continually. Of course, after one perfects the art of hand-balancing so that it can be done by muscular feeling only, he may perform it blindfolded; but this ability comes only after years of practice, and until it is developed the balance is very uncertain when the vision is uncertain.

Why is it that a golf player who, after becoming proficient in that pastime and who can break one hundred almost at will, will perform rather amateurishly once in a while? I, myself, have found it to be very provoking that on certain days when I feel that I can duplicate my previous game I play like a dub. Gymnasts also frequently have their off days.

These experiences will occur repeatedly in any athlete's or physical culturist's life, and when they occur it is best not to attempt one's full program for that day but wait until the next day or the day after, when one again feels in A1 condition. I really believe that many boxers lose their titles because they ignore this fluctuation of energy and box on days when they are off form. Boxers who have beaten their opponents on previous occasions sometimes will be knocked out in turn by the same opponents. This, of course, may come from over-confidence and carelessness, yet I believe that in most cases it happens simply because the boxers experience the off day that anyone will experience occasionally in his athletic career.

Peace of mind and harmony play an important part in endurance. If there be cares or worry upon the mind it is impossible to accomplish what ordinarily can be done when the mind is carefree. More nervous energy can be wasted by worrying or brooding than by any other drain upon the body. I remember reading, years ago, about Joe Gans, the colored lightweight champion, who publicly announced his secret of losing weight in order to make the lightweight limit. In short, he just worried about losing. Whether this be practical or not remains to be seen. I know, however, that anyone who worries will become thinner, and if the worry is continued nervous exhaustion very likely will result.

If one desires to develop endurance, he must develop organs and nerves capable of withstanding enduring or continued activity. This necessitates the avoidance of every influence that will weaken the organs or lessen the store of nervous energy, and every influence that hinders normal functioning of the organs, normal response of the muscles, and normal transmissions of energy, over the controlling nerves when the energy is required. Not only must worry and adverse thoughts be avoided, but every physical healthpromoting and health-sustainng factor must be adopted and a rational program adhered to. Furthermore, a definite goal must be kept in mind, efforts must be always in the direction of that goal, and nothing must be allowed to bring doubts or at least to continue doubts of ultimately reaching that goal.

V

PHYSICAL activities come under two headings—one is exercise or recreation and the other is work or labor. You often may wonder why a laboring man, performing his daily toil, does not develop into a great athlete. He surely performs more repetitions throughout the day than any physical culturist will ever attempt regularly to do. Would it not be logical, therefore, to assume that all these muscular efforts would produce enormous muscles, great strength, and almost tireless energy? If we look deeper into the physical condition of laborers we find that not one in a hundred possesses a symmetrical development. The laborer is strong, it is true, and his endurance powers are excellent, for I am sure neither you nor I could undertake to bend our backs the number of times a day that the average workman does in the performance of his duties. Yet he is easily defeated in practically every physical encounter with a trained athlete.

In the first place, though his muscles are larger than the average man's they are so accustomed to being used in the same restricted manner that they are almost helpless when required to be used in a different way, especially if the different way be a complex way. His back may be exceptionally strong, much stronger than the average athlete's when it comes to bending; yet the average athlete easily can outlift him in all feats of strength where the back is brought into play. In spite of the endurance he possesses from performing movement after movement, day after day, the average laborer would make a poor showing against a trained wrestler, boxer or runner. It is only by working slowly and relaxing between movements that he is able to keep up his daily toil for eight hours or more at a stretch.

Now let us consider the athlete. Uusually he exercises for but about fifteen minutes to an hour a day. This time is spent either with the weights or gymastic apparatus or in

36

calisthenic exercises. He works with enthusiasm, and fair rapidity throughout his entire exercising period. At the completion of each series of movements each muscle is tired, sometimes almost to the point of exhaustion; but when his drill is finished he feels in tip-top condition and like whipping his weight in wild cats. For the remainder of the day he relaxes, so far as special exercising is concerned. During this period of relaxation his muscles are given a chance to recuperate and grow. His muscles are trained by daily exercising to work in coordination, each helping the other. It is only natural for him to endeavor to excel in one or more of various sports, whether they be jumping, running, weight lifting, wrestling or boxing. He will find that his muscles will enable him to excel in these sports far above the average man, assuming that they have equal theoretical knowledge of the sports undertaken.

Pit the laborer and the athlete together in any sport whatever, and, even though their knowledge of the sport is equal, the trained athlete will come out winner on every occasion. Why? The answer is that during working hours the laborer has been working too hard, overworking his muscles and denying them the chance to build up to the degree of muscular coordination such as is possessed by the trained athlete, who relaxes most of the day. Work wears out the one while exercise strengthens the other. The laborer works for necessity, but the physical culturist exercises for recreation and to gratify his enthusiasm. The physical culturist would be no better off than the laborer if he exercised excessively, for he thereby would bring on exhaustion and overwork, just as does the working man.

A well-trained body is first of all essential to anyone interested in endurance. It would be folly to take a man who has never run more than a block in his life, out for a two- or three-mile trot. In the first place he could not last— he would collapse far from the finish. And if a man who has never exercised in his life were compelled to go quite a distance for something which must be gotten hastily to save someone else's life, it is doubtful whether the patient would survive. The man would not have the endurance nor the strength to carry him through.

I remember reading years ago, when I was a boy, about Bob Fitzsimmons, who was then heavyweight boxing champion of the world. I think it was back in 1897. He was at the bedside of his sick wife, and the doctor told him that oxygen must be administered immediately to save her. Fitzsimmons ran at top speed, late at night, from block to block, looking for a drugstore, hospital, or police station where he could get an oxygen tank. At last he found one and carried a tank of oxygen while running at almost the same speed back to his home. His wife was kept alive. If Fitzsimmons had not possessed a well-trained body and the ability to run rapidly and long, which he secured from doing his road work prior to his fights, there might not have been this story to tell.

Therefore, the advantages of a well-trained body readily can be seen in cases of emergency, whether it be in the performance or duty for others or to save one's own life. To begin with, the exercise enthusiast, in addition to having greater strength, naturally will have more coordination in his movements than will the average man, who lacks experience in physical training. The untrained man possesses little, if any coordination. In fact, instead of coordination there usually will be found muscle antagonism.

It is amusing to note how clumsily a beginner will dance. You can see them on any dance floor. Yet, the simple steps of the Charleston, foxtrot or waltz are easy after a little practice. Have you ever noticed a woman throw a ball? Of course, she has little cause to do so, but when the attempt is made it plainly can be seen even by the inexperienced that something is wrong, for none of the muscles concerned with throwing the ball seem to work in unison. Anyone who frequents a swimming pool will see how clumsily the beginner endeavors to learn the first rudiments of any stroke, and yet swimming is easy after one learns how. How amateurish the experienced boxer will make an inexperienced one appear. No matter what sport or pastime or walk of life you may consider, the inexperienced man or woman puts forth twice as much effort in the beginning, and this effort is clumsy and awkward, because of the fact that instead of muscular coordination there is muscular antagonism—some of the muscles opposing those doing the work actually contract instead of relax, thus hindering the action and doubling the effort.

No one can appreciate muscular coordination more than the weight lifter or the golfer. The weight lifter must stand "just so," grip the bell properly, time his movements accurately, and, when bringing the bell overhead, lower the body downward at the exactly required moment. The golfer must be in perfect form for his drive. He must work in unison from the top of his head to the soles of his feet. The slightest movement will have a tendency to displace the center of gravity of the body, thus interfering with the stroke being made, whatever its nature.

The only way to obtain coordination is by practice; and by practice I mean to exercise. In animals coordination is instinctive; but in man it must be developed. Everyone has observed the movements of a cat. They are graceful and harmonious, and yet no one ever taught a cat how to move. For a human being to obtain the grace of movement of a cat it would, undoubtedly, take years of practice. A pianist requires considerable practice before he is able to place his finger on the key he desires to strike, but when he is able to do so he does it with no less effort than a chicken expends in snapping its beak at a grain of corn.

When one masters the art of coordination, if it may be termed an art, he really possesses what might be termed muscle sense. Have you ever watched an experienced tennis player? If you have, you have noticed the wonderful dexterity with which he returns the serve or volley. He sees the ball coming toward him but he does not see the ball hit the racket. His judgment and muscle sense know just where and how to place the racket to hit the ball and he does not see the ball again until it has rebounded quite some distance away from his racket. Those of you who have played handball will appreciate what is meant by, and the importance of, this sense of coordination. I know from my own experience in playing handball, especially in a four-wall court, that the ball shoots around the walls with such rapidity that it would be almost impossible for the eye to follow its progress. But my muscle sense allows me to realize where the ball is about to come and, naturally, by putting my glove in the right place and adding a little force for the return serve, I am able to stroke the ball and control it, sometimes, of course, better than at others.

Magicians have proven to the public that the hand is quicker than the eye. But the hand or arm, as in handball or tennis, must be much quicker than the eye; for if one took the trouble to turn the head, even though slightly to allow the eye to follow the ball, he would lose control of the return serve. In baseball the batter depends a good deal upon his muscle sense; and even though his eye sees the ball coming toward him, yet, as in the case of handball and tennis, his eye does not see the ball hit the bat; but his muscle sense and judgment enable him to swing the bat where it will meet the ball—not timidly but with tremendous power, and with almost uncanny certainty, as with Babe Ruth and some of our other home-run hitters.

Last year I received the honor of becoming an Honorary Member of the Mounted Police Association of New York City and also of the Honor Legion of the Police Department of New York City. One of the requirements of the initiation was for me first to ride a mechanical horse and later a live one. I am almost ashamed to admit that I am an amateur at equestrianism. Of, course, through my athletic abilities I had but little difficulty in mastering the rhythm of the mechanical horse; but when it came to find the gait of the live one I was all at sea. The bumping I received during this initiation on the live horse I painfully remembered for many days afterward. Now, if I had possessed the muscle sense gained through practice in horseback riding, I would not have been black and blue from this seemingly severe initiation. Even though I since have taken up horseback riding seriously, still my endeavors at my first attempt must have been just as amusing to those who knew how to ride, as are the antics of a fat man in a gymnasium for the first time.

Muscle sense really is the feeling we have of the force with which a muscle contracts and in the direction in which it acts. Without it we would not be able to place our hand or foot at the exact spot which we wished to touch. Muscle sense involves the antagonistic muscles as well as the muscles used in directly in performing the movement. These antagonistic muscles must be worked to act in harmony and coordination with the other muscles before muscle sense can be perfected—the opposing muscles must be fully relaxed so that the acting muscles will be completely unhindered while they are performing; but when the need arises the muscles must be able instantly to reverse their condition and relaxation. This muscle feeling or sense can be gotten only by practice and experience; and if one never has attempted any pastime or sport it would be ridiculous for him to compete against anyone but a beginner like himself.

Undoubtedly one of the most striking examples of muscle sense is that exhibited by the juggler. Juggling requires both dexterity and balance. Many times I have attended vaudeville shows and have seen almost unbelievable stunts performed by these master jugglers. I remember one man in particular who juggled a chair, a pail, a coat, coat rack and hat—five entirely different objects of different sizes and weights. He threw them into the air and turned them around, and caught them again without dropping one. Surely his eyes could not clearly see all these objects. Therefore, he depended wholly upon his muscle sense to gain the applause of the audience.

The pianist must eliminate all stiffness from his fingers before he can expect to excel with his chosen instrument.

Stiffness, if not due to some inflammatory or structural change, would indicate that the extensor muscles were interfering with the flexors. If the oarsman allowed his triceps to interfere with the pulling power of his biceps when rowing, he would not make the speed he is after and he would soon tire in the arms should he be attempting a long row.

The same thing applies to any muscle or group of muscles in the body. If the flexor and extensor muscles interfere with each other's action, it will be necessary to put forth several times the effort and energy in order to accomplish any performance. That is one reason why laborers cannot compete with the experienced student of physical culture; their muscles have been exercised in their work in a restricted manner, and there has been no coordination for refined or complex movements.

The reader may wonder what all this has to do with endurance; but I am working up to the application. I am endeavoring to prove to you, and I will, that complete control of the muscles, which includes coordination and muscle sense, must be gotten first of all before you attempt anything in the line of endurance exercise. The man who properly exercises his muscles will, first ol all, keep fit and he always will have his muscles under his command, the same as a general who continually drills his troops, has them under command.

So many would-be physical culture enthusiasts forsake their exercising in disgust just because they experience muscle fever or a feeling or exhaustion the day following their first workouts. If such enthusiasts would use a little common sense and judgment and begin systematically, their attitude regarding physical development would be entirely different. A baby first crawls, then walks, and then runs. As gracefully as a cat may be, a new-born kitten is very clumsy. Everything must progress, and it is impossible to progress beyond the laws of nature. It is true that some progress more rapidly than others; but this is because some learn coordination, muscle sense and the art of relaxation much sooner than others, just as with two individuals taking piano lessons together one will make better progress than the other.

VI

To A BEGINNER in physical training, fatigue is the first discomfort or pain experienced, whether he is standing before a mirror performing dumb-bell or calisthenic exercises, or whether he participates in open-air sports, such as rowing, jumping, games, or what not. He finds that after a very short period of exercise he is out of breath and some part or other of his body seems incapable of further movement. An aching is experienced, indicating, of course, that the muscle has been used to the limit of its power of recuperation. Usually after a short period of rest he will be able to resume activities. But if a beginner allows his muscles to reach the aching point or if he resumes exercise before fully recuperating after he has become fatigued, he will learn to his sorrow the next day that he should have exercised less strenuously. The lameness he will experience will prove very uncomfortable, and if more than one group of muscles should be affected he is liable to find himself in bed, suffering from muscle fever.

This reminds me of one of my pupils who came to my office one afternoon and enrolled for my course. I outlined about five or six exercises for him to follow for the first few days, to get his muscles in condition for a few of the more vigorous movements, as he had never before done any exercising. I particularly told him to take it very easy and not to exercise more than about five minutes for the first day, and after a day or two he could increase this period by a minute or two. I told him to come back and see me within a couple of days. When the time came for his second visit, this pupil "showed up missing"; but about a week later he lagged into my office, pale and in a half-alive condition. Upon asking what had been the trouble he told me he had exercised for five hours the day after he enrolled. He further stated that the next few days after that he had spent in the hospital. Well, no wonder! Evidently my instructions to him to take it easy had gone "in one ear and out the other," and his enthusiasm to become suddenly muscular and strong overwhelmed his sense of good judgment—if he had any!

If by chance you are one of those who have taken no active exercise for a few months and then return to a gymnasium, you may find at the outset that you still retain all your old pep and vigor. You can perform all of the most difficult movements and with nearly the same ease as you used to, and you may work in the gymnasium the first time for the same length of time to which you have been accustomed in the past. In the evening, however, a little or, perhaps, a great weariness and sleepiness most likely will come over you, indicating that your body craves more sleep than usual. But sleep may not come for a long time. If finally you fall asleep, you probably will awake shaking and perspiring. Your tongue may be coated and your appetite lost and your limbs will be trembly. These are the symptoms of muscle fever, which is a type of poisoning resulting from an excess of the waste products of muscle contraction and nerve action.

After a while, however, the fever will decline, but you still will feel uncomfortable and your muscles will feel the need of rest, and for several days thereafter they will be sore and stiff. All this happens when one has exercised strenuously after a long lay-off. However, stiffness or muscle soreness does not occur always in the same manner. If the exercises you take, which you have not practiced for some time, are confined to local or single muscle groups, instead of experiencing muscle fever you will experience simply a severe lameness or muscle soreness in the localized areas that took part in the exercise. This soreness will last about the same length of time as if you develop muscle fever.

To you who have exercised, wouldn't it seem foolish for someone who had spent years at a desk and who had taken no exercises whatever, to be entered in a one-mile run against experienced competitors? What would you think of him—of his judgment, and of his chance of winning? After the first block or two you would soon express your opinion in mirthful gestures. Yet this very same inexperienced man, in his own heart and soul, will feel he is capable of defeating the others, at least holding his own with them.

Nearly all my life I have been interested in the boxing game, and whenever there is a good boxing exhibition I make it a point to attend if at all possible. I have seen fighters grow up, so to speak. I have watched their interesting wares in the preliminaries, and have seen them progress month by month and year by year until they have reached the top. Also, I have seen these same first-class boxers retire after losing their laurels, and nearly all of them were much below the age of thirty when their crowns were lost to others. It is pitiful to see some of these retired boxers, whom the public classifies as old-timers, return to the ring to combat against youth. Probably financial need may be the first thought; but surely a prominent thought must be that of their ability to defeat the newcomers just as they, themselves, defeated all comers in their own heyday. But youth must be served, and the poor showing of the old-timers brings nothing but comment and boos from the audiences.

While all this apparently may have little to do with the subject of endurance, the few illustrations given will help to bring out my points. There may be a great many other conditions largely governing the ability of the one-time champion boxer, such as reduced recuperative power, lack of judgment in distance and timing, etc. He ignores these, or does not estimate their extent, and his intentions and thoughts are just as serious as those of anyone else who thinks he can make good without first giving serious thought to his physical preparedness, which directly and deeply concerns endurance.

In my high school days I played halfback on our football team, and even in those days I considered that I was in good condition, for I always had been interested in physical training. Without question I was the strongest boy in the school, because I was the only one who exercised faithfully. Others may have been mildly interested, and probably performed their exercises spasmodically, working a day or two and then dropping it for a week or so. My excellent condition made me over-confident. We had a tough team to play, and after memorizing the signals I really felt that I did not need to go through all the minor practice in which the rest of the team indulged. They practiced running, tackling, passing, punting, etc. My teammates probably respected my condition, for—without being boastful—I had made good on previous occasions the year before. Finally the day of the game came; and I played with my usual enthusiasm. But for the next day I was so lame and muscle sore in nearly every part of my body, it seemed, that I actually was feverish. I was learning the lesson each and every one must learn, by painful experience, who does not heed the warnings of others more experienced in physical training and sports.

Stiffness or muscle soreness need not generally follow vigorous work which tires the muscles quickly. Sometimes you may be misled into thinking that you are exercising with sufficient ease to prevent soreness and that you have discontinued the movement before any signs of fatigue set in. And, at other times, an exercise can be pushed to the limit of your powers without the slightest disturbance following. This is because stiffness depends rather upon your general and muscular condition than upon the manner in which you perform the work. For instance, a moderate exercise, such as walking, may result in stiffness in a man accustomed to complete inactivity, while running or jumping will not produce any disturbance in the well-trained man.

I very seldom have had a real massage after exercise. I usually massage myself with a coarse towel by friction, in the form of a rubdown. Should I exercise too violently at some new sport or pastime to which I am not accustomed, and should I experience muscular soreness, I generally treat the condition with hot applications and gentle massaging with my own hands. It may be that I do not mind muscular soreness, as I have been exercising for so many years that I suppose I am somewhat used to it.

But not long ago, while I was in the best possible physical conditon, I chanced to meet a masseur whose reputation travelled before him. This masseur had been praised by many for his remarkably effective, magnetic manipulations. Having some leisure time on this day I decided to try one of these famous massages. I must admit that the masseur knew his business; he understood anatomy thoroughly, which is essential to the proper manipulation of the body. Whether he made extra efforts because he knew who I was —and probably a hard-boiled critic with a chip on my shoulder—I do not know; but I must admit that I felt better mentally, if not physically, afterwards. Now mind you, I said I was in the best physical condition at the time. I had been training daily month after month and without growing stale; my muscles never had possessed better contour; nor had my vitality and strength ever been greater than on this day. Yet, the next morning my muscles were stiff from my neck to my feet.

I surely enjoyed this experience, for it furnished me with further proof that even though the muscles have been accustomed to performing heavy or even tedious movements, still by offering them such a slight change it was possible to bring on muscle stiffness. It proved that the muscles can be deeply affected by manipulations; but I doubt very much whether such manipulations would increase their size even a fraction of an inch, even if they were massaged daily. Rather, I would say that a gentle massage to muscles not in the best possible condition might enable them to perform more vigorous contractions afterwards, and muscles in perfect condition can be benefitted by a gentle massage, which undoubtedly will somewhat help them, also, in performing endurance work.

What effect has massage beyond its chief effect of increasing the circulation? It produces heat in the muscles— the same as is acquired by the contractions and extensions of the muscles in active exercise. There must be a certain temperature before the muscles can act in harmony and coordination, for cold muscles are practically as useless as are the muscles of a man in the declining years of his life.

Even though the student feels that he is in full command of all his physical powers and that he has superior quality of muscle, it will be well to consider here the subject of improvement of muscle quality.

Heat plays a very important part in governing the quality and usefulness of a muscle. When a muscle is cold it naturally becomes somewhat stiff and this experience can be had by anyone who is exposed to a brief exposure in winter when improperly clothed. One seems to shrink together, so to speak, and a sort of numbness overtakes him. If he were to attempt to perform a certain feat, no matter how simple it might be, such as jumping, running or the like, he would find that he would experience more or less pain in the muscles involved.

This brings to mind a personal experience which happened one summer a year or two ago on the beach. It was a cool day with a strong wind blowing. I had been in the water for some time and naturally I felt chilly when I came out. I started doing hand-stands on the sand in order to warm up and increase my circulation. After doing a dozen or more hand-stands with various forms of push-ups, I suddenly decided to turn a back handspring. I did, and something snapped in my left ankle. All the blood had been centered around the muscles used in handbalancing, and my feet were cold and not in condition to receive the force when I landed on them somewhat heavily. I limped around for about nine weeks with a sprained ankle, the penalty of my folly; but I since have made it a point never to attempt any movement or stunt that requires skill or strength, before first seeing to it that my muscles are warm and in proper condition for that particular work.

When you attend a track meet you will note how the sprinters always warm up before the race. They trot up and down, either stationed in one spot or in short jogs here and there on the track, in order to get or keep the muscles of the legs warmed up and in condition to compete. If a runner did not do this he soon would find himself far behind his competitors.

Heat is an indispensable element for muscle contraction. However, if the temperature rises too high, then the heat destroys the activity of the muscle. This easily can be illustrated by anyone who desires to experiment with hot bathing. After lying in a tub of very hot water until one is perspiring profusely, one will experience a sleepy feeling, probably a "dopey" feeling, rather than one of energy. If, however, this hot bath is not too long continued and is followed by a cold shower, one will regain activity of the muscle, because the cold water restores normal temperature and at the same time shocks the nervous system and acts as a stimulus.

Heat can be produced by excessive muscular work as well as by bathing and other external means, and such muscular effort can overheat the blood and poison the nerve centers, doing considerable temporary or even permanent damage.

It readily can be seen, then, that heat, or warming up of the muscles, and placing them in a condition to do work is just as important as is practice in any sport which will produce muscle sense, and as important as training that will develop muscular coordination. These are among the first rudiments of physical training that the student must acquire before attempting anything in the line of endurance work.

In the production of heat, diet plays a very important part. The athlete who does not eat properly and whose food does not properly proceed through the process of digestion, will find himself lacking in muscle condition and, therefore, in his endurance efforts. The body is entirely built up from the materials drawn from the food we eat; and certain physical and temperamental characteristics depend considerably upon where one lives, because of the variance in foods native to different geographic regions, especially different zones. The foods grown or produced in a zone as a rule are best suited to the needs of the natives of that zone. The Eskimo and the inhabitants of the far North must eat a fatty diet or foods that will produce considerable heat. Whether they understand the food question or not seems to make no difference, for they evidently are concerned only about their tastes and the gratification of their appetites, and these in all cases call for heat-producing foods, in the far North. The people who live around the Equator subsist on an entirely different diet, and they could not tolerate by taste or digestion, the food eaten by those in colder regions.

Again bringing in one of my own personal experiences: I have lived in the tropics and I have lived in Alaska. I even have had the good fortune to be within a few hundred miles of the North Pole, where, as far as I could see, there was nothing but pack ice. Do you suppose for one instant that the fresh fruits and green vegetables I ate in the tropics would be sufficient for me in a temperature far below freezing? In the North I continually craved greasy stews, thick soups, potatoes and the like, and the reader can rest assured that, while eating with my coat collar up around my ears, such food tasted better to me than any ice cream soda ever did when the thermometer registered over one hundred degrees Fahrenheit.

To show what effect food has upon the body, just go without a few meals and experience the pangs of hunger. You will find that you will not be very much inclined to exercise when your stomach seems to be begging for nourishment. A man who regularly performs violent muscular work cannot furnish the quantity of heat needed by this work after a two-day fast.

Practically, it is impossible to outline a definite diet that everyone may follow regularly. The constituion of each of us is different from that of others. The nervous individual needs far different food than does the phlegmatic person, and the large, tall man naturally will require a larger quantity, owing to the size of his organs, than will the small-framed, shorter man. Each one will have to experiment for himself; and as there are so many varieties of foods to select from, I am sure it will not be difficult to find the proper diet. It may be necessary for one to make a fairly careful study of some of the magazines or better books dealing with the subject of diet, in order to learn some of the principles of dietetics. The subject of diet has received much thought in recent years and almost any recent book on the subject will give many valuable sugges tions for the man who exercises. Personally, I believe in variety. I do not think a man should, unless there is something organically wrong with him, stick to one exclusive diet, for the body requires all kinds of foods. I believe, however, that it is far better to secure variety from meal to meal or from day to day, rather than to have a wide variety at each meal.

I have done considerable experimenting with diets. I have lived exclusively on milk for a while. I have tried raw foods. I have tried milk and eggs; and I have tried the mixed diet—meat and vegetables. And, although I must admit that the vegetarian diet seems to be most satisfactory, still there are times when my body seems to need a thick steak; and when it does I believe in satisfying the needs of my body. Too much meat, of course, will prove harmful, as will too much of any good thing.

Whatever foods are selected as best serving one's individual needs, it is essential that one's digestive organs and the organs of elimination function properly in order to produce the proper heat for the body. As stated before, without this proper heat, coupled with muscular coordination and muscle sense, no one will be able to perform endurance movements to any marked degree.

The student must bear in mind that when seriously considering endurance work, or any exercise that requires an extra expenditure of energy, he also must increase the quantity of his food. By this I do not mean to overeat or to stuff oneself to capacity; but unless the diet is somewhat enlarged or at least has additional nutritive food values added, he will be continuing his exercising not on physical strength but on nervous energy. It is a common occurrence for an athlete to continue in his sport or pastime without experiencing fatigue while performing endurance work and yet steadily lose in weight. This, however, cannot go on indefinitely. He must look into and adjust his diet and way of living, or he soon will be burning the candle at both ends; and he is liable to decline into a condition of such diminished resistance that he no longer can defend himself against the numerous injurious influences which react upon him from without, just as a man who is run down from a cold may be susceptible to any disease with which he comes in contact.

But to return again briefly to muscle stiffness. Before undertaking endurance work the muscles must be prepared by training so that stiffness does not develop. The best procedure for preventing stiffness is to do a small amount of work every day and progress according to your vitality and inclinations. Of course, if one follows inclinations alone he is apt to find himself becoming lazy, for it is natural for all of us to endeavor to become as comfortable as possible at all times. But habits are easily formed; and as we all are more or less victims of habits, it is an easy matter to form the habit of taking exercise at the same time each day, just as you eat your meals at the same times or do many other things at regular times during the day.

VII

ABILITY brought on by practice, endurance, fatigue, and recuperative powers all are closely linked together. No one can make good, whether he be a runner, boxer or athlete in any other sport, unless his organs as well as his muscles work in harmony, and unless the muscles possess the ability to recuperate between exercises. A beginner's muscles will sadly lack these qualities, and largely because of the lack of acquired coordination through overcoming the antagonistic muscles. Naturally, in' such a condition fatigue sets in.

Often deer chased by huntsmen have been known to drop dead from exhaustion; but during exercise a human muscle never reaches the condition of absolute fatigue or complete powerlessness. This is prevented by the painful sensation experienced before the muscle becomes absolutely incapable of action. The rest that is enforced by the thoroughly aching muscle checks the further development of fatigue. Even should the enthusiast desire to continue the movement after the muscle is aching, the pain and suffering soon would become so intense as to eliminate all forced action by will power.

I once read what was an excellent illustration proving that muscles really never became absolutely exhausted. It also was stated that all the will power a man may possess cannot exhaust the last remaining power still left in a muscle after it reaches the severely aching point. As nearly as I can recall it, it read something like this: One of the most tiring attitudes to assume is that which consists of holding the arms outstretched horizontally. The deltoid or shoulder muscle does most of the work. There are very few who are vigorous enough to hold the arms in this manner for more than five or six minutes. At the end of this time the deltoids cannot act any longer and the arms drop. But the muscles are not exhausted; the fibres still possess a great contractive force. This can be proven by the fact that certain stimulants, such as electricity, can bring into play this motive force over which the will no longer has any action. If by waiting until the sensation of fatigue becomes unbearable to a man who is holding out his arms, and if at the moment when he declares he has used up all his power and is about to let his arms fall, you apply a strong electric current to the shoulder muscles the fatigue and feebleness seem to vanish and the arms remain outstretched, showing that the muscles had not lost all their contractile power. It is undesirable to work a muscle to such a degree that an abnormal stimulant is required to bring forth further contractions. It is wise to discontinue the movement and to relax when, or even before, the aching point begins to develop. After a time it will be found that you will not have as many aches as you used to have, and these, of course, are eradicated by practice and experience in the various movements and by the development of better tone—better endurance—in the muscles themselves. The more experience you have in a certain movement the more endurance you will acquire. Do you think for one instant that a mountain climber could continue until he reaches the summit if it were his first attempt? Naturally, the first time he climbed anything he would experience fatigue; but by constant practice he finally is able to avoid this fatigue by having his muscles in condition and working in coordination.

One year while in Seward, Alaska, I stood gazing at quite a high mountain on whose round top there had been placed a flag. I inquired of a passerby for what purpose the flag had been put there. He told me the mountain was known as Marathon Mountain, and that each year there was an annual race up to this flag pole and back, the winner being presented with a prize. I almost opened my mouth in astonishment, for it was hard to realize how a human being could run up the side of such a heavy grade and for so long a distance, for this mountain must have been fully four thousand feet in height. If any one of you has tried to run uphill you will appreciate the wonderful endurance it takes to run the short distance of even one hundred yards. I feel quite certain that those who participate in this annual Marathon Mountain run would not think of making the attempt without first rehearsing at least a good distance up the slope, and regularly, for several or many days before the race.

Anyone who wishes to experiment in uphill running should try running two or three steps at a time up the stairway of a tall office building. I am sure he would find himself extremely tired long before reaching the top, and I would not recommend such exertion to anyone who has not conditioned his legs, heart and lungs beforehand, by first practicing one flight, two flights a few days later, and progressively to the top in this manner. It would be foolhardy for anyone to attempt it otherwise; for not only would fatigue set in, but the heart action would be greatly disturbed, possibly the heart damaged, and most likely serious consequences would follow.

The power to resist fatigue is essential in acquiring endurance, and, in fact, may be said to constitute endurance. If you have refrained from exercise for some time and your body suffers for the want of it, fatigue well may be dreaded; whereas, if you exercise daily and keep your body in good condition you will have no cause to dread fatigue. But by having too long periods of repose, such as omitting your exercising drills for days at a time, it will make you more susceptible to muscular fatigue and muscle lameness than if you daily performed physical activities for but a few minutes. Therefore, it is essential, as I have so many times stated, always to be in good condition.

The only way to gain the power to resist fatigue is to increase power and endurance of muscles, heart and lungs. You must continue each day whatever exertions you are performing, until the muscles begin to feel tired. After a while what exertions once brought on fatigue and demanded relaxation no longer will do so. In time you can continue with the activity without thought of fatigue, and for what, to the inactive person, will be an almost unbelievable length of time.

A well-trained man resists fatigue easily, not because he ignores the painful sensations which usually or frequently accompany work, but because these sensations are not produced in him, or at most are produced in very slight and easily variable degree. Exercise induces nutrition in all the tissues of the body. This makes them more resistant and firmer, and, in a sense, arms them against shocks and friction and protects them against the accidents of work. On the contrary, prolonged repose makes the tissues softer and more susceptible to the shocks and accidents.

Fatigue in all its forms is felt especially after too much rest has been taken. If anyone has had the experience of traveling across the country, from coast to coast, he will realize more than ever the value of daily exercise. I have taken this trip numerous times and, while I always keep myself in excellent condition, a threeor four-day ride on the trains, with its dusty or super-heated atmosphere and lack of activity, makes me feel, upon arriving at my destination, that my energies have been lowered appreciably.

Once, after I had been in heavy active training for several months, I went from New York to Seattle, Wash. After leaving my baggage at my hotel, I took a walk up and down the hills of various streets. Anyone who has been to Seattle will know what steep grades there are along some of the side streets which cross the main thoroughfares. I found in time that upon reaching the tops of these little hilly streets I was beginning to puff, when ordinarily I would not have been so affected by such exercise. This breathless condition was brought on by my four-day train ride, during which I had practically no physical activity whatever. This indicates the importance of allowing no day to elapse without doing exercise in some form or another.

My belief is that in these modern times the automobile takes a great many years from any people's lives. How many business men are there who upon leaving their homes walk to the elevator of their apartment or hotel, which carries them down to the street and there awaits their car, which brings them direct to the office where they again enter an elevator, which brings them practically to their desk?

After a day of inactivity they ride home; and they repeat this same routine day after day. It is no wonder they become fat and flabby, with absolutely no endurance. They would suffer from lameness and stiffness if they walked the length of two or three blocks. Finally they wonder what their troubles may be. Perhaps, upon advice from their physician, they decide upon an hour's walk. They probably are in bed with fever the next morning. But take the postman, who walks and stands continuously all day long. He goes to bed without feeling any ill effects from the exertion, and awakes in the morning feeling fully fit for his duties.

The fatigue which follows an exercise of speed is unlike that experienced after an exercise of strength. In performing strength work the muscular contraction is well in evidence and is slow and prolonged, and the fatigue is especially felt in the muscle. The limbs become weary and congested. The blood flows to them and swells them, which is usually the most encouraging thing a physical culture enthusiast can experience. When I first began exercising, I performed my work before a mirror, and I was just as enthusiastic about my measurements and increasing the size of my muscles as my pupils are today. I actually measured my muscles every day to see whether or not they were increasing in size. How encouraged I felt when, upon finishing a certain movement and measuring the muscle which performed the movement, I found that it had increased about one-quarter of an inch in size; and how disappointed I was when later in the day I found I had lost the one-quarter of an inch, as the blood had left the muscle, naturally decreasing the size of the muscle. But the constant swelling up or bringing of blood to the part used by the activity of the exercise positively will increase its size permanently, if not overdone to the point of exhaustion of cells, energy and building material. But more of this later.

The expression "nervous fatigue" gives a good idea of the kind of disturbance which easily is recognized by those who have ever prolonged an exercise of speed. There is less desire for sleep, and the appetite also lessens. These effects are produced by the great expenditure of nervous energy, which an exercise of speed makes necessary and which makes the repair of the exercised structures more difficult. Speed work, also, will take off weight, which can be laid to the expenditure of nervous energy in performing the speed work, just as any nervous strain upon the body is bound to reduce the weight.

While fatigue may be muscular or nervous, it also can be mental and take the form of depression. This depression can be created by overwork and by using the will power to force the muscles beyond their natural tiring point. It is interesting to note what stimulating effect the mind has upon the muscles, especially when they are fatigued. Those who have engaged in actual warfare know what aching and swollen feet mean upon returning from the trenches, exhausted and depressed because of the tremendous amount of nerve force and muscular action used in advancing and in retiring in combat. It is a common sight to see comrades dropping exhausted, one by one, on their return march. But let someone shout, "the enemy is coming," and everyone will be on his feet, forgetful of fatigue and depression.

It will be seen, therefore, that besides our will power forcing our muscles onward, that additional stimulus can be created by fear and excitement. Of course, greater reaction is bound to follow when such added stimulus compels further muscular action. But whether it be fear of bodily injury or fear of losing out, such mental stimulus will prove very interesting in the study of endurance work, which I shall discuss in another chapter. It is not wise to force the muscles by the will to such a degree as is possible by some emotion unless a life or a great accomplishment depends upon it; and except in some crisis or urgent need it is well to discontinue movement when the feeling of tiredness enters the muscles involved. Muscles should be in such condition that fatigue would not manifest itself, through training and possessing the ability to recuperate between movements. And again let me repeat there probably will be lack of recuperative power if relaxation between movements is not secured, or if coordination is defective and muscle antagonism plays the chief role during the movements.

The sensation of fatigue prevents one from having an exact idea of the energy which the muscular fibres still possess; and it compels rest long before all the force of the muscles has been spent, just as hunger warns us that we need food long before the body becomes weakened from lack of nourishment. The sensation of fatigue should put us on guard. As I have said, it would be dangerous to continue working until the muscles become completely exhausted and incapable of contracting, and we should look upon early signs of fatigue as nature's warning to discontinue all movement.

The student will find that a greater number of movements can be made if the mind centers on other things. If you think about what you are doing the concentration on the movement naturally will tire your muscles quicker than if your mind wanders. Mental concentration while exercising, therefore, can be seen to be better for muscle building than for endurance work. As an organ, the heart is an example of this. It beats throughout our lives. Its movements are involuntary, just as are the movements of the lungs. Neither the heart nor the lungs ever determines the sensation of fatigue in individual muscles or groups of muscles.

The muscles ordinarily under the control of the will have the same immunity to[s] fatigue if their contraction is made more or less involuntary. This easily can be observed in patients suffering from St. Vitus' Dance or those suffering from palsy. In either case movement after movement is performed against the will, from morning till night, and yet muscular fatigue does not develop in appreciable degree. If an athlete were to continue such a series of movements, impelling him to do so by force of will, complete exhaustion would set in before many hours would pass.

The student will find for himself that an exercise which is accompanied by concentration, that is with the thought on every movement he is doing, will prove more fatiguing than a movement which is performed independently of the will. Again may be mentioned the beginner with his lack of coordination and muscle sense and who is wholly dependent upon his enthusiasm and desire to achieve in a difficult sport or pastime. The tension he puts forth with each effort can be likened to the most strenuous muscle building work for the experienced athlete.

VIII

I HAVE brought out that good lungs are essential for endurance. The one who has the best "wind" usually wins the long distance or long drawn out event. As you know, the essential condition of breathing is the presence in the lungs of air and blood. The oxygen in the air purifies the blood that is pumped by the heart through the blood vessels. However, this is physiology, which can be found in any book on that subject; and those who have read my book Here's Health will find complete answers to questions on physiology that may arise in their work.

Have you ever found yourself within sight of the railroad station and afraid of missing your train? There probably was a quarter of a mile still to go and your watch showed that there was less than two minutes till train departure. You rushed to make it. For months you had been accustomed to use the same gait, perhaps, in walking to the station. However, in this instance you have had to pluck up courage and run, or else wait for the next train. Perhaps you were in fairly good condition—your legs quite strong.

However, after a few seconds a peculiar distress came on. Your breathing became difficult and your chest felt heavy. Mayhap you caught the train, but what happened after you entered the car? As the train started you sank almost exhausted upon the cushions. In spite of the fact that your exertion had ended, your distress continued. For some minutes you were out of breath—winded. You may have been surprised when you considered that though your legs were strong yet your lungs or heart appeared weak. Your legs did the real work, why didn't they feel the fatigue first? But every time you work your legs you also give your lungs and heart an added amount of work; and in endurance tests it is these organs that first feel the strain, in those who are unprepared by graduated systematic and regular exercise.

I am a firm advocate of deep breathing and giving the lungs plenty of work. The more often you take deep inhalations through the day the larger your rib-box will become and the greater will be your lung capacity; but deep breathing alone, while sitting, walking or standing, will have no direct increasing effect whatever upon endurance. If you desire to possess wind—that staying power that will enable you to reach your goal in endurance activities— you must go through the actual practice in the sport in which you expect to excel. Deep breathing taken at various intervals throughout the day will, of course, help considerably in increasing capacity and strength of the lungs but it will not bring you endurance.

I doubt whether anyone has a better lung capacity than most opera singers. They have mastered the art of breath control and are able to breathe so systematically yet unconsciously that it in no way interferes with their singing; in fact, their ability to breathe properly makes possible their superior singing. They are able to hold their notes for an astonishing length of time. Yet they would make a poor showing in any form of endurance work if they have never practiced that particular activity.

While attending normal school, studying to become a teacher when I first became interested in this work, I frequently played handball and squash with one of the Metropolitan Opera House bassos. Now, handball is a game that will "wind" one very quickly unless he becomes proficient in this pastime. By becoming proficient I mean experienced in the practice. This basso (whose name is immaterial here) appeared to be in excellent condition. His shoulders were broad, his body erect, and he possessed great depth to his chest. His arms and legs, also, had pleasing curves, which indicated that he had kept himself in excellent condition by some form or other of exercise. But he had done no running, and it was evident to me, after playing one game of handball with him and watching him pant for breath, that all the exercising he had done consisted of movements performed while standing stationary. He probably had squatted up and down for his thighs, rose up and down on his toes for the muscles below the knee and swung his arms to and fro, possibly with Indian clubs or dumb-bells, to develop his upper body. He was sadly in need of endurance work. Perhaps such work did not appeal to him, and as musicians and singers seem to live in a world of their own, perhaps he felt that endurance would not better in the least his singing ability.

Breathlessness is a general effect—a result of the total quantity of work performed by the muscles used in an exercise. On the other hand, muscular fatigue is but a local effect. It is localized and in direct proportion to the share in the work taken by each muscle used in the exercise. When the work is too light to produce breathelssness, it can produce fatigue if your effort is performed by a small group of muscles or by groups of very weak muscles. But if your exercises involve a great number of muscles or are performed by large muscle groups, the effort you put forth will be too great to produce local muscular fatigue and, therefore, you will find yourself breathless—winded. Breathlessness is caused partly by the over-driving of the heart, and by the congestion of the lungs which this immediately produces. When you perform an exercise calling for a maximum or prolonged effort, you will find that breathlessness comes on with astonishing rapidity.

As I stated previously, if you run upstairs you will find breathlessness occurring much sooner than when you run on the level ground. In certain muscular actions fatigue takes the form of breathlessness, and the respiratory distress forces you to stop exercising long before the muscles themselves are fatigued. You can swing your arms, for example, or exercise with light dumb-bells, following the oldfashioned dumb-bell drill, and continue until your arms are aching, and yet you will not be winded. This explains why a well-developed man, whose shoulders are broad, whose deltoids are rounded, and whose pectorals and upper arms have beautiful contour, may not necessarily be any good when it comes to endurance. He may have developed his upper muscular body without developing his lungs. But, if this same muscular individual has firm, well-rounded thighs and well formed muscular hips, you can rest assured that his lungs are in A1 condition; for it is practically impossible for one to perform vigorous leg movements without bringing into play all the "wind" or lung power and capacity that he possesses.

Try the simple experiment of holding your arm out sideways. You will find that after about four or five minutes you will be compelled to lower it, and yet your breathing will be normal. Try the same exercise, holding in your hand a pair of three-pound or five-pound dumb-bells; still, even after your deltoids are thoroughly aching, you will find your breathing about the same as before you began the test. You may be obliged to stop these light upper-body exercises, not because you are out of breath but because your muscular or nerve force has been expended.

An authority on exercise once heard a horse trainer say, "A horse trots with his legs and gallops with his lungs." This expresses well the importance of pace in the production of breathlessness. Why should a horse be more out of breath after a gallop than after a trot? The first thought would be to attribute the more prompt breathlessness to the greater swiftness, but we must not become confused between pace and speed. You can slow down the gallop of a horse until it falls behind another horse which may be trotting. There are some horses, as you know, so awkward that their gallop is as slow as a fast walk. However, no matter how slow a gallop may be the horse will become out of breath quicker than he would from an equally rapid trot. This is because more muscles are used at the same instant, the movements are more rapid even if the pace is not, and the entire weight is lifted from the ground at once, very frequently.

Therefore, one does not become breathless under the same conditions as produce local muscular fatigue, such as exercising the muscles singly, tiring the biceps alone as by curling, or the deltoids alone as by raising the arms sideways. It is true that it is impossible to exercise the arms, for example, without working the shoulders, the back and the chest to a considerable extent. Even though you concentrate wholly upon arm work, the muscles of your back and shoulders will be exercised to some extent by the arm movement. In spite of this, you will find that your muscles will tire long before you become winded. If you want to see the difference between twenty-five movements performed by the muscles of the upper body and twenty-five movements performed by the muscles below the waist, just do any exercise you may choose for the muscles above the waist for twenty-five counts and then jump as high as you can twenty-five times without stopping, and note the difference in your breathing after these two exercises.

The peculiarity in the breathlessness caused by heavy leg exercises is not that it is hard to inhale, but that it is hard to exhale all the air from the lungs. No better instance of this can be had than in swimming. It is a very easy matter when swimming the crawl stroke to inhale as much air in one gulp as is needed; but you will find when you turn your head sideways for your next inhalation that, unless you are an expert in the art of breathing, all the air will not have been exhaled from your lungs and you cannot inhale much. This breathing difficulty is one reason why very few of us care to become long distance swimmers. Breathing while swimming is an art which must be mastered, and there is not one swimmer in a hundred who has fully mastered it. These are the ones who swim a mile or two with small effort and at the end find themselves breathing just as normally as when they started.

Upon investigating the condition common to all muscular activities which are said to be capable of rapidly producing respiratory troubles, you will find that all movements that require a great expenditure of force produce breathlessness. Of course, breathlessness can be produced by holding the breath, and anyone who has endeavored to swim under water for any distance realizes when he has to come up for air that he needs it badly, also that he is somewhat winded. This is a voluntarily created breathlessness. I would not advise anyone to see how long he can hold his breath, for such a willful respiratory disturbance interferes with the heart action, circulation, and general health.

The condition of the extensor muscles of the thigh, and the other muscles of the legs as well, have a good deal to do with the wind. For instance, if you trot at a certain rhythmic pace, let us say for a distance of a quarter of a mile, you will not be as winded as you would be if, while keeping the same rhythmic pace, you sprang higher into the air or put more effort into each leg movement. In other words, the more effort placed upon the leg muscles, the quicker you become winded, even though you do not change the timing or the pace. This is because the greater effort greatly increases heart action and circulation and makes a greater demand upon the lungs for oxygen to take care of the larger quantity of blood passing through them at a more rapid rate. More nervous energy is used, and, too, the interest usually is more deeply aroused when one is undergoing more rapid exercise. These all affect the wind.

Another illustration is deep knee-bending exercise. You can squat and raise for, perhaps, one hundred or more repetitions before you feel slightly out of breath. (I am taking it for granted, of course, that you are in good condition.) Just try and do the same exercise but, instead of simply raising the body by the strength of your thighs, push off the ground vigorously and jump into the air. You will find that your respiratory organs will feel the effects of these latter efforts much sooner than the former.

To determine for yourself which of certain movements produce local fatigue and which movements produce breathlessness, sit on a chair and rotate your feet around in circles until the muscles of your shin become paralyzed from fatigue. This is an example of local fatigue. Next have someone sit on your shoulders or else have a bar-bell resting on your shoulders, and perform the squatting exercise; that is, bend your knees until you almost sit on your heels, and then rise again until your legs are straight. You will find after a comparatively few number of repetitions that you will be breathless, because you have used larger muscles strenuously in groups. You have worked the thighs, the calves, the back, and even the abdominal muscles in the performance of these movements. If you desire to develop endurance, it is much better to perform exercises that produce breathlessness than it is to carry out movements that simply produce local fatigue.

If you exercise the muscles singly, that is one at a time, until each one is thoroughly tired, you may develop them; but they will lack coordination and the muscle sense that will be required in performing endurance work. On the other hand, if you exercise the muscles in groups, you naturally induce breathlessness much sooner, but at least you are working them in harmony and coordination, and at the same time you are increasing your lung power, which will be needed in all endurance pastimes. In one of my other books, Muscle Building, I have gone into this matter in detail.

When an exercise causes breathlessness it is not wholly due to the contraction or usage of certain muscles or the disturbance of certain organs during the exercise. It is due largely to the excessive expenditure of force which the exercise necessitates. Breathlessness occurs whenever muscular work produces in a given time more carbonic acid in the blood than the lungs can eliminate in the same time. The quantity of work necessary to produce breathlessness, then, will not be the same in all persons, for all cannot eliminate from the lungs the same quantity of carbonic acid in the same length of time. Therefore, in order to avoid becoming breathless during an exercise you must regulate the work of the muscles by the eliminating power of the lungs, in such a manner that the quantity of carbonic acid produced in a given time shall not be greater than that which the respiratory organs can dispose of during the same time.

Naturally, a man or an animal will adopt a pace in running from which he cannot materially depart without producing breathlessness. If a fairly violent exercise is performed continuously for an appreciable length of time, breathlessness always is produced in the end, even though the individual does not exceed his natural pace. If, for example, you can run at a moderate pace for five minutes without losing your breath, you will find breathlessness occurring in a quarter of an hour, even though you do not change your pace in the least. That is because, even though the work you are doing remains the same, the demand upon the lung power will become greater by the continuance of the movement, and the circulation of the blood through the lungs becomes increased.

A beginner in taking a cold shower usually makes plenty of noise. The shock of the water suddenly striking his body compels him to gasp for breath, and his respiratory organs are forced to undergo considerable activity. After a while, however, he becomes used to it and, of course, in time his body will require a greater shock to produce the same respiratory activity as occurred when the water struck his body early in this experience.

Every violent physical sensation, wherever situated, will react upon the lungs, just as any powerful emotion also will make its influence felt. Every time the rhythm of breathing is much disturbed, breathlessness is produced, even when you may be in the condition of muscular repose. The observing student will find that if his mind is disturbed by worry or the like while going through his exercising, breathlessness will come quicker than if his mind were at ease.

It readily can be seen that another essential point toward endurance is composure of mind. Worry will bring on fatigue quicker than anything else. If, while performing movements, you are worrying about the form in which you are doing them or are thinking too much about the muscles involved, you positively will tire much more rapidly than you would if you mentally relax, the only thing on your mind being your destination or goal.

An excellent illustration showing how breathlessness will hinder your physical activity can be gotten from anyone's own life. How many times have you become provoked at someone? Unconsciously your fist may have clenched and you had a "chip on your shoulder," so to speak, ready to begin hostilities at any moment. You may not have observed it, but if you will recall the way you felt, you will recall that there was great interference with your breathing. The mental disturbance acting upon the general nervous system in that case produced respiratory disturbances.

Many people are greatly affected by shock, a sudden shock causing such a state of breathlessness as to make a person more or less gasp for air. There is a striking resemblance between the respiratory disturbance due to a violent moral impression and that which results from a powerful physical sensation. The man running, the man under a cold shower for the first time, and the man overpowered by fear, experience a kind of shock in the region of the nerve centers which preside over the respiratory movements. Therefore, in order to acquire endurance you must have the respiratory system working in perfect order, and not easily disturbed by various influences. The mind should be free from emotional disturbances, and there should be harmony of thought.

The one chief difficulty experienced by endurance athletes is breathing; and especially, strange as it may seem, the exhalation of the air. If during a run you keep the same rhythmic pace, you will find that more steps will be taken while inhaling than while exhaling. This is the case if you are breathing naturally. But after you stop running you will find just the reverse—the exhalations will be longer than the inhalations.

Those of you with experience in weight lifting will know this only too well. I have attended many contests in weight lifting and in some have acted as a judge, and, therefore, have had ample opportunity to observe the various physiological results from this pastime. I remember that while acting as a judge in one contest a strong man who possessed a very powerful build performed the lift of "two hands anyhow." This lift consisted of raising an enormous bar-bell to arms' length overhead with as many stops between the floor and straight arms overhead as the lifter desired to make. He first brought the weight to the height of his knees, and rested the bar thereon by slightly bending his legs. Next, with a tremendous heave, he brought the bell to the upper part of his thighs and held it there, while assuming a slightly squatting position. With another mighty heave he brought the bell to his belt line, there resting it on the belt and securing it in the fatty folds of his abdomen. The next tremendous effort brought the bell to the height of his shoulders and there is was locked by the strength of his arms and balanced on his upper chest. During each one of these series of lifts he took a deep inhalation and had to hold his breath during each ascent. Finally, with a mighty upward jerk he pushed the bell upwards about a foot or so, quickly bending his knees and ducking under the weight and then standing erect while holding the weight at full arms' length overhead. After balancing it there for a moment he let the bell drop heavily to the floor, and while doing so the air came out of his lungs with a roar that could be likened to the gushing of an oil well. His respiratory system was affected for a short time afterwards and his breathing was done under difficulty.

Here is an example of effort in practically only one feat of strength performed, yet the nervous concentration, plus the physical exertion, created breathlessness, while the entire performance was of not over one minute's duration. Every exercise which demands a series of efforts at short intervals for even a short period of time very quickly produces maximum effort of the heart and possibly fatigue of that organ, and affects the respiratory organs.

IX

BY THIS TIME it is evident to the student that before he considers endurance he must acquire muscular coordination, muscle sense, and good wind, and have his organs functioning properly. A youth may possess all of these qualifications, but how about the one who has slipped backwards? He is the fellow I am trying to reach, and if I did not think I could fully arouse his interest before the time I finish this book, if I did not hope to convert every reader to the fact that he must continue to keep himself in good condition and not backslide physically, and if I did not think that you who read this book would feel that I am correct in claiming that everyone should be able to save his own life, in most emergencies, I would cast the whole manuscript into the ocean, whose waves almost are touching my feet as I write.

For one who has discontinued training, it is advisable to begin very lightly and progress just as slowly as if he had never before had experience with exercising. In this manner there will be only a slight discomfort showing on the following day, which can be worked off by gentle movements in order to improve the local circulation and carry off the retained muscle waste, as well as to avoid over-work. It is a fact that too much exercise is more harmful than none at all, as in the case of the circus strong man.

It is folly to compel yourself to exercise when the body says "No." Just when you receive this warning, you alone can tell. But there is a distinct difference between the call for rest and relaxation after having had enough, and the sluggish feeling of indolence. How many times have you, who have had experience with exercising, gotten out of bed in the morning with sleep still in your eyes. It seems at such times as though you could scarcely open them. It may come from the fact that you were up late the night before. In most cases a cold bath soon will remove this feeling and give you the desire for working. But should it not do so and you still lack the starting energy, it will be much better for you to skip your morning exercising period on that day. If you cannot perform it later, take none at all that day, and the following morning will find you prepared and fit to tackle a vigorous drill.

If you fail to follow this plan you are liable to overwork your muscles, and overwork would be a case of fatigue being pushed to the extreme. Overwork also can be produced by continuing an exercise or a sport after your good judgment and bodily feeling tell you to stop.

Have you ever attended a six-day bicycle race? Perhaps many of you have. Around and around the saucer track the riders go. These men have wonderful endurance powers, brought on, of course, by their continuous riding in six-day races throughout the year. The first day or so finds them still fresh, but if you can get close to them when they dismount from their wheels, after relief by their partners, to carefully study their faces, you will find that haggard, drawn expression on each of them, signifying the drain upon their energies. They are overworking themselves, and if it were not for the vast amount of sleep that each six-day rides takes when the race is over, they soon would find themselves physical wrecks.

The reader must not misunderstand me and think, when I am emphasizing the fact that everyone must possess a certain amount of endurance, that I am advocating for him marathon running, six-day bicycle riding, or twenty-fivemile endurance swimming, for such is not the case. I want simply to impress upon each and every reader that a fair amount of endurance is absolutely essential not only for safety's sake in saving one's own life and the lives of others, but for anatomical and physiological reasons as well. Endurance exercises, if not carried out to the extreme, positively will prolong life.

Overworking of the muscles burns up the tissues faster than they can be replenished, with the consequence that instead of the muscles becoming larger they grow smaller and smaller in size. This is proven by most endurance runners. You would think anyone who runs mile after mile would increase the size of his legs from such prolonged effort, so that eventually they would attain enormous proportions; but the fact that almost every endurance runner has thin legs proves that the work or pastime in which they excel breaks down the muscle tissues faster than they can be built up. Hence, in endurance work an abundant diet is essential.

Only the other night I was attending a boxing show, and among the various celebrities introduced from the ring was a tall thin fellow, whose height I should judge to be about six feet, but whose clothes hung so loosely upon his framework that he appeared rather ungainly. Much to my surprise, this young man was introduced as a champion runner, he having run without stopping for one hundred miles. He was introduced from the ringside that night for the announcement that he intended to run seventy-five miles the following Saturday. It was hard for me to imagine anyone running one hundred miles without stopping, and yet this youth accomplished the feat; so seventy-five miles would not prove very difficult for him. But I wondered, and I presume there were hundreds of others whose thoughts were the same, why he did not possess a massive chest and Herculean legs. But it is the same with him as it is with practically all other endurance athletes—the longer they work, the thinner they become.

Exceptions to this rule can be had in swimmers. It seems that the water creates a fatty tissue around the muscles of most swimmers. It is nature's way of protecting them from the cold, just as the people of the North usually are stouter than those living around the Equator. As all rules seem to have exceptions, it is well to look into the better nutrition of long distance swimmers. You all have noticed on the bathing beaches how the thin man suffers as soon as he comes out of the water. His teeth chatter and he presents a woeful sight. You often wonder why he does not dress instead of endure his shivering. It may be that the stout people naturally take to the water and, therefore, can stand the cold much better than the thin ones. You frequently see the stout man play around in the water and on the beach, sometimes for hours at a time, and not seem to be affected. Probably this is the reason why stout people naturally become distance swimmers after they have perfected the art of swimming.

Approaching exhaustion will manifest itself not only in the muscles themselves but in the organs as well. The heart will beat with exceptional rapidity and force and the respiratory organs will be greatly affected. Prolonging an exercise beyond this point might cause serious complications—heart strain being the most serious one. The heart is a muscle and, therefore, is enlarged through activity. It develops thicker, heavier, stronger walls; and in the athlete it propels the blood more vigorously than the smaller, weaker heart does in the one who never exercises. Excessive exercise, however, induces wearing and degeneration and diminished strength of the fibers, producing dilatation of the cavities of the heart resulting from a thinning, weakening and stretching of their walls. Usually the athlete who strains his heart is "through." Therefore, my earnest advice to all my readers and pupils is to make doubly sure not to prolong a movement beyond the point when they feel a degree of fatigue that is slight enough that the exercise could be continued for some time longer.

This feeling of fatigue will become less and less pronounced as one progresses with the work. Suppose, for illustration, one feels slightly fatigued after performing a movement one or two hundred times. After this same movement has been performed for a week or two, it will be found that two hundred times does not cause fatigue; an additional twenty-five to fifty repetitions will be possible before experiencing this feeling. A similar illustration may be gotten from running. Suppose one is able to run a quarter of a mile before the respiratory apparatus is affected or the heart begins to thump. It won't be long before it will be possible to run half a mile before experiencing the same functional disturbance of the organ.

To cite from my own experience: when I first became interested in swimming I used to find great enjoyment in swimming in pools. To swim the length of the pool, which was sixty feet, seemed to be sufficient for me for some time. The exertions I went through in those sixty feet left my muscles tired, my breathing equipment exhausted and my heart beating rapidly. This was because I was a beginner. It was not long before I was able to swim two and three laps and upon completion of the additional lap or laps I would feel just about as tired as I did previously at the end of one lap. After a year or so I was able to swim a mile without as much organic disturbance as I had in the beginning after my first lap's swim.

This shows how progression can be made naturally, without any strain upon the organs. If in the beginning I had attempted to swim two laps, the over-exertion may have exhausted me to such a point as to strain my heart. Or a little later, when I was able to swim three laps, if I had forced myself to swim four or five laps the same serious condition might have resulted. And today even though I am able to swim considerably more than a mile (though I am not a professional long distance swimmer), if I were to force myself to swim three or four miles, should it be possible for me to do so, serious organic disturbances might ensue.

Mental depression or indisposition must not be mistaken for exhaustion. By this I mean that if you are performing work or a sport that you indulge in more through necessity than through liking, often a mental disturbance manifests itself and you imagine you feel tired long before you actually do.

There may be some requirements in exercising that you will need to make good to perfect your body to a condition of physical independence, so to speak—to a point that will give you courage and a self-satisfied feeling when you realize that you are fit and able under almost any ordinary circumstances to protect yourself in emergency. If you should experience unpleasant exercises, such as forcing yourself to swim under water a certain distance or working up to a point of being able to swim half a mile or more, your thoughts may tell you to stop long before you feel slightly fatigued in the muscles used.

You may wonder why I dwell so much on water sports; but I really consider swimming the foremost accomplishment in anyone's life from the standpoint of self protection, at least. I really believe there is not one person in ten who is a good swimmer. The five or six of the ten who are able to swim or to keep afloat will be incapable in case of emergency, and the remainder who do not know how to swim at all will be absolutely helpless in emergencies in the water. Expert practical knowledge of swimming has saved many a person's life. But though you may be able to swim on the surface of the water for a reasonable distance, you have only about fifty per cent, of the knowledge necessary should emergency arise. You should be able to swim a reasonable distance under the water, also. While this may be disagreeable to many, and difficult as well, owing to the holding of the breath and the presence of mind required as to sense of direction, still for life saving it is absolutely essential that this be mastered. Suppose you should be cast suddenly from a ship into the ocean or lake or river; the weight of your clothing would not be an asset toward keeping you afloat. You may find your head under the water on numerous occasions. You may be compelled to unlace and remove your shoes while keeping afloat; and you will find that taking off a pair of shoes while floating requires your head to be under water many times before you successfully remove them. Each time your head is under the water, you must hold your breath to prevent the water from entering your lungs. Unless you are accustomed to swimming under the water, you are liable to become panicky and drown.

When I was a small boy we all used to swim in the Harlem River. We did not bother with bathing suits, and would have much fun diving. I recall how muddy the water was, but that made no differnce to us; we liked it just the same. The diving stunts we performed then we would not attempt to do today, for we have better judgment. I often recall of diving twenty or more feet into three feet of water. I had to turn quickly upon reaching the water, to prevent ramming my head into the river bottom, and still my chest and abdomen would scrape the bottom. As we grow older such foolhardy stunts never enter our minds except as memories.

I recall that on one hot summer day, while diving off one of the piers, a number of us went off at the same time. We all came up and climbed back except our friend Joe. We were not very uneasy because we knew he was an expert swimmer as well as diver; but we looked about for him, thinking he might be playing a trick on us, hiding somewhere underneath the pier with the intention of sneaking up behind us to push us into the water. We waited and still no appearance, and finally Joe's head came up out of the water, directly alongside a barge which was near the spot where we were diving. I recall the agonized expression on his face. He told us afterwards that he started fetching, or swimming under water, and when he came up for air he found himself underneath the flat-bottomed barge. It seemed almost unbelievable, but still fresh in my memory is his recital of his miraculous escape.

Think of it—when coming up out of the water for air, to find yourself underneath a large flat-bottomed boat! He simply had to turn around under the water and continue swimming underneath the barge until he saw the water becoming lighter from the reflection of the sun. Then he knew he was safe. His head and lungs seemed almost bursting, and it seemed impossible that he could hold out long enough to escape.

I frequently see this boy, now grown, and a few years older than myself; and many times we have looked back on the days when we were boys and often mention the narrow escape he had in the Harlem River. If he had not had presence of mind, plus the ability to hold his breath and swim some distance under water, he would not be alive today.

This is one true and excellent proof of the value of being "at home in the water." Of course, I do not believe in one endeavoring to see how far he can swim under the water, or to the point where he begins to feel distress in his lungs or heart. But this distress first manifests itself in the mind; and the desire to give up too soon never will enable you to swim the distance you should be able to swim in proportion to your size, organic condition and swimming ability. You will find, when you feel indisposed and inclined to come up for air while swimming under water, that if you repeat several times to yourself, "just one more stroke," you will be able to take half a dozen or more extra strokes, possibly without any ill effects organically. You alone must be the judge as to your respiratory condition. If when under water your lungs feel like bursting, you have remained under too long for your good, though no real and lasting harm may result from an occasional experience of this kind.

One year while in southern California I took the boat to Catalena Island. From this island tourists are given the opportunity to ride in a glass-bottomed boat, through the bottom of which can be seen the sea-growth and shells and fish to a depth of about thirty feet, for the water is unusually clear. The lecturer on the boat I was on was in a bathing suit, and after explaining the different sights which we saw as the boat glided along, he announced he was going to give an exhibition of under-water swimming and he asked all to take out their watches to time him, to see how long he could stay under the water. I would not have believed it possible had I not timed him with my own watch while he was under water; but when he came up it showed that he had been under almost four minutes. A truly remarkable test of what might be termed breath endurance, or lung capacity.

However, holding the breath and working at the same time may cause dilation of the heart. But I think everyone should progress to the point of being able to swim or hold the breath under water for at least one-half to threequarters of a minute. This, of course, must be worked up to, for to endeavor to hold the breath for one-half a minute in the beginning, if it were possible to do so, might be dangerous.

X

IN ORDER to perform endurance work the art of relaxation must be mastered. There must be no more tension than absolutely necessary in any part of the body, particularly in unused parts, and antagonism of the muscles should be absolutely absent. In the first place, in order to acquire relaxation one must perform movements slowly. If rapidity of motion is indulged in, it will be found impossible to relax, for the thought stimulus necessary for performing movements rapidly tends to keep certain muscles ever in a state of tension.

The human body can be somewhat likened to an engine. The engine keeps running so long as fuel is supplied; but the body differs in that, in spite of the most nourishing diet, muscular movement becomes impossible after a certain period of exercise, and the work is necessarily stopped. The human machine can work only intermittently. Relaxation is required, because of the need of repair by the living organism. The more a machine is used, the quicker it will wear out. The automobile, for example, can run only for a certain number of miles before it becomes useless. A cannon is good only for a certain number of shots. But the human body is quite different; the more work you give it, within reason, the better condition you place it in, and the stronger one becomes.

Rest is the essential condition for the elimination of waste products of work, for during rest the formation of these waste products is lessened and those that have been formed during activity are taken up from the cells and discharged from the body. Rest also is essential for the repair of the organism, because during rest the processes of assimilation, by which repair takes place, is not hindered by the processes of tearing down, which goes on so actively during exercising.

During sleep and relaxation the loss from the tissues in the performance of exercise is restored. The more strenuous the exercise, the greater the loss sustained and therefore, the more relaxation and rest will be required for repair to be completed. A person who does not receive his proper amount of rest is carried on by nervous energy, and he does not give his tissues a chance to recuperate as nature intended them to.

Relaxation, then, is necessary so that the organs may repair the losses they have suffered during the period of activity. If it were not for this period of relaxation the body would not undergo repair but quickly would be worn out from the work. Every time you exercise a muscle you will find it swells up. That is because the blood rushes to the part used. Cells are destroyed. If you prolong an exercise and do not receive sufficient relaxation, the muscle will wear away instead of becoming stronger and larger.

Relaxation is just as important to the athlete as is exercise, though, of course, relaxation without exercise will not make the athlete. Exercises that cause breathlessness rapidly naturally do not need the same length of relaxation afterwards as is required by movements which bring on breathlessness slowly, such as endurance work. Exercises of endurance cause fatigue less quickly than exercises of speed, but require longer periods of repose, because the fatigue is more general and results from a prolonged draft upon the nervous energy. An energetic man can walk five or six hours without relaxing, but he will find that when fatigue does come on slowly it also is slow to disappear. The same thing applies to the distance runner, swimmer, rower, or participant in any sport or pastime requiring a great number of repetitions of movement.

In your experience with exercising you undoubtedly have overworked sometime or other. If you recall the stiffness and lameness that you experienced for several days afterward, this will serve to indicate the length of time required for relaxation after a prolonged workout. It is impossible for one to go through the strenuous movements he went through the day previous after he has exercised sufficiently to produce stiffness and soreness. On the other hand, you many times have performed vigorous, heavy work until after only a few movements you were panting for breath, yet after a minute or two of rest you were able to proceed. This shows the difference between the different forms of work and indicates the length of the relaxation period required by each.

If the boxer did not have one-minute rests after each round he would not be able to continue with his endeavors during the next three-minute round. During the one minute of rest his breath and his muscles receive relaxation and he is appreciably restored. One minute of rest to three minutes of fighting is sufficient for the trained and younger man. But as one becomes older he does not recuperate so quickly, and naturally one-minute rests prove insufficient. I fully believe that the experienced boxer in the thirties could easily defeat all the comers in their teens if his body could recuperate as quickly as theirs during the one-minute rest periods between rounds. It cannot and that is why youth must be served in the ring.

Relaxation may be secured in different forms or by different methods. It is not necessary for the runner to lie flat on his back in order to relax and recuperate from the exertions of a long run. When he walks he finds ample rest for the muscles, heart and lungs. A swimmer does not need to get out of the water after he has been forced to swim until tired. He is able to obtain relaxation by changing his stroke or speed or by floating on his back with but very slight movement of the fingers or feet. In many other activities it is possible to secure sufficient relaxation for rest of all muscles and organs by merely reducing the severity of the exercise or shifting the work to other muscles. However, when one is thoroughly fatigued or has any distress at all, a complete rest by reclining is safer.

So many times I have found myself with limited time to exercise. I usually allow one hour each day for my exercising period, which includes bathing and dressing; but many times I have had but thirty minutes for a workout, and on these occasions I was compelled to rush rapidly through the work. I did not feel like skipping certain exercises which I had been doing with a definite purpose in each morning's drill. Therefore, I had to hasten from one exercise to the other, with practically no "breathing spell" between exercises. Of course, I did this from choice and not from necessity, for whether or not I had skipped a few of the movements would have made very little difference. But all of us have hobbies, and it is my hobby, when I select a certain routine to follow for a few months before changing it for another routine, to carry out my program in every detail as I have outlined it for myself. During these rush periods, as I call them, I rest one set of muscles while I work others. For example, I find it does not affect my respiratory organs to exercise the muscles of my legs (calves) or my neck. Therefore, after violent arm exertions or thigh exercises I find relaxation by performing neck work or calf work, and yet at the same time I am continually in motion.

The above suggestion might prove valuable to a busy man, but I give it only to show that relaxation can be had, though not complete, in other ways than lying down or sitting at repose. Sleep, of course, is complete repose, because in this condition all the muscles usually are relaxed and the organs work with less energy, and that is why sleep and the proper amount of sleep are essential. A person's sleeping hours should be regular, for sleep plays just as important a part toward the performance of endurance work as does wind, coordination, muscle sense, and relaxation. To the one interested in endurance, there is nothing better as a means of storing up energy in order to perform or accomplish his purpose than a good night's rest before a contest.

Have you ever seen a fat man on a hot day stretched out in an easy arm chair? He seems to be in a state of complete repose, and usually he is. But observe the thin individual. Instead of sitting comfortably in the chair, he seems to be always fidgeting about, turning or twisting occasionally, and keeping himself under some tension at all times.

Have you ever noticed the complete relaxation of a cat when sleeping? If you were suddenly to grab a slumbering cat you would find that no matter what part you touched, apparently without any force it would twist or bend from your hand or fingers because of its complete relaxation. Try this degree of relaxation yourself the next time you feel like flopping, so to speak, in a chair. Are your legs crossed or is your arm supporting some weight of your body? Or are you in a state of complete repose? Only in the latter can you rest and recuperate fully.

We all should learn the art of relaxation, for it will prove a valuable asset during our endurance efforts, or at any other time, for that matter. Suppose you wanted to take a pair of five-pound dumb-bells and curl them alternately with each hand to your shoulder. If, for instance, you wanted to make four or five hundred repetitions you would not go at it vigorously, but you would let the bell drop to your side after each flexion, and you naturally would perform the movements in the easiest way possible. Not that I advocate the use of light dumb-bells for four or five hundred counts, for I believe it to be a waste of time and energy to do so. But the method is similar to anything you may undertake in the form of endurance work, and which you should be able to perform in securing the preparedness for saving your own life or that of someone else. If you were rowing a boat and had to row for two or three or more miles through heavy seas, I am sure you would not go at it so vigorously that your arms and shoulders and back would become tired after a few hundred strokes with the oars. You would not even grip the oars tightly. Instead you would row the easiest way possible and after each back stroke you would obtain as much rest and relaxation as the brief seconds allowed.

A man I know told me an interesting story of his experience during the late war. The ship of which he was one of the crew was torpedoed by a German submarine and all hands were thrown into the sea. Very few survived, but he was one of the fortunate ones in a rowboat containing three or four others. Although the sea was calm at the time and he was an experienced oarsman, still he and the other men were forced, when a breeze sprang up after a few hours, to keep the boat cutting through the waves for over thirty-six hours before they were picked up by a passing ship. Only his previous experience with rowing enabled him to perform this wonderful endurance feat, for his companions were almost useless to him so far as assistance was concerned. Two of the men were thrown overboard, having died from exposure during these two cold North days. (They also were without food and water.) Although the shock caused a reaction on this man shortly afterwards, still today he is perfectly well, thanks to his endurance. His knowledge of rowing was no different from that of anyone else, but he knew how to relax between strokes; for if he had not relaxed, his body would have collapsed long before the boat was picked up by a passing ship.

Give the average physical culturist a shovel and direct him to dig a deep hole somewhere. In about fifteen minutes his hands will begin to show blisters. But a day laborer, who works from morning till night, does not hurt his hands by holding the spade. The laborer most likely does not possess as much energy as the physical culturist possesses. He merely has a thicker skin, brought on by the constant friction and pressure incident to his occupation. This illustrates what changes may occur daily in the organism under the influence of work. Just as the skin of the hand undergoes changes from the continual gripping and handling of the spade, so every organ undergoes a material change from the indulgence in exercising.

Let us return to the ringside. How many times have you watched the boxers pummel each other with all their might? You have seen them land terrific body blows, and yet after the resounding thud of the glove on the side or abdomen of the opponent, you seldom see a mark left by this impact. Oftentimes the boxer hurts his own hands in delivering the blow more than he hurts his adversary. If this same boxer landed these blows on a beginner, you would find the latter's skin not only black and blue but abraided as well. The explanation is that the well-trained boxer no longer feels a blow of the fist, as his flesh has become so hardened that it is not injured by the impact.

Exercise does not merely harden the skin and the muscles; it consolidates or makes firm all the organs as well. I frequently have illustrated the difference between the race horse and the truck horse in referring to human beings. The race horse is always "on edge"; he performs light, speedy work and, therefore, remains thin; whereas, the truck horse performs heavy slow work and, naturally, becomes "beefy." Animals that do hard work acquire tough and solid muscles and tendons, and the same condition of these tissues develops in human beings who labor or exercise heavily. Perform slow movements and you will become heavier and more muscular; exercise in a nervous, light way and thinness will be the result. That is one reason why weight lifters always are "beefy" in appearance, as well as strong, while boxers, runners and track athletes, who do lighter work, usually are of the more slender, wiry type.

To produce the same physiological effects upon the body, work done in an exercise of speed must be equivalent to that performed in an exercise of strength. One hundred repetitions with three-pound dumb-bells, for example, may produce the same amount of breathlessness as ten repetitions with thirty-pound dumb-bells. In other words, the amount of exertion spent in these two exercises balances, and equal breathlessness develops because equal energy has been expanded. A man who slowly goes upstairs carrying a heavy weight on his shoulders is doing a work of strength, while a man running as fast as he can along a level road is performing an exercise of speed. Both of them do a great quantity of work in a very short time, one by slow movements, each representing a great expenditure of force, and the other by often repeated, rapid movements, each of which represents a very much smaller quantity of work but which in total cause a considerable expenditure of force. Therefore, an exercise of speed can lead to an accumulation of work equal to that done in an exercise of strength.

In an exercise of speed, just as in an exercise of strength, there develops what is known as a thirst for air. This thirst for air is to the lungs what the appetite is to the digestive organs. The difference between exercises of strength and exercises of speed is that the former produce a condition of muscular fatigue before breathlessness, whereas, the latter produce breathlessness before muscular fatigue. Suppose you take hold of a one hundred-pound or one hundred and fifty-pound bar-bell—the weight depending, of course, upon your strength. You hold this bell in front of you, both arms relaxed, and then bring it to the chest in what is known as the two-arm curl. You can perform this movement, let us say, about ten to fifteen counts, when you find that the supinator muscles of your forearm and the biceps of your upper arm are beginning to ache. Upon lowering the bell to the floor you may take one or two deep inhalations, but after a few seconds' rest you are able to perform another movement with the same barbell and tire some other part of your body. Now, suppose you run at top speed for a fair distance, say one hundred or two hundred yards. You will find at the finish of this sprint that the muscles of your legs are just warmed up, and if called upon to perform additional movements they would be capable of doing so. But what about your wind? You are "puffing" considerably. The exercise is one of speed, and quickly produces breathlessness.

An exercise of strength also can be made an exercise of speed; but this would be termed forced exercise and, most likely would prove quite harmful to the heart.

About a year or two ago I had the pleasure of meeting one of America's foremost athletes, who came to visit me in my office. Being inquisitive by nature, I inquired into his methods of development and training—what routine he followed. He told me that he worked as rapidly as he could with heavy weights, going from one exercise to the other without rest. He did not relax during the whole period of his drill, which consumed about twenty minutes of time. To my mind it was a truly remarkable case of forced exercise, for here he was performing strength work and at the same time speed work.

For experimental purposes, I tried it myself on the following day. I used the same amount of weights as he told me he was using; did the same number of repetitions and with the same speed; that is, I went through practically this young man's entire drill in the same time that he did it. The reader must bear in mind that, though I always keep myself in excellent condition, upon following this routine, I found that my respiratory organs were greatly bothered and my heart was pumping with unusual rapidity. Undoubtedly, this was caused by performing the exercises in a different way from which I had been accustomed to doing them. The difference in ages between this young man and myself should be taken into consideration. He was twenty-one while I was thirty-seven. Nevertheless, it proved to me that such forced exercise was apt to cause serious organic disturbances. I would not suggest that anyone attempt such experiments unless he is positive he can endure them; and when breathlessness overtakes one he should not force the exercises against his organic capacities. I am still convinced that relaxation and breathing periods between exercises are of the utmost benefit and necessity to the physical culturist who takes pride in his health, condition, and appearance.

Exercises of speed increase the activity of the respiratory organs with much less fatigue of the lungs and heart than is created by strength exercises, owing to the absence of forced muscular effort. Such effort occurs only accidentally in exercises of speed, but is compulsory in exercises of strength. But exercises of speed will not develop the bulk and strength of muscle as are developed by strength work, for there is a smaller supply of blood forced into the muscles during and after speed work; therefore, the nutrition of the muscle is less active during this kind of work. It is a physiological fact that the nutrition of any part of the body is in direct proportion to the quantity of blood with which it is supplied. But while exercises of speed fall short as developers of muscles, they are much better for the internal organs and they increase the size of the chest and lung capacity—effects of great health importance.

Speed work naturally requires more concentration and more power of will in the perfomance of the movements. There also is an increased expenditure of nervous energy in the performance of this work. Speed work produces greater "irritabilty" (responsiveness) in the muscles than any other forms of exercise. This irritability of muscle enables it to act quicker at the command of the will. If you go into a gymnasium and observe the different athletes exercising, you undoubtedly will notice the difference in irritability of the muscles in the various individuals. In some persons rapidity of movement seems to be natural, and you see how fast they move and how quickly they perform their various stunts. Then you will observe how slowly others go through their exercises. Their muscles seem to be very slow in obeying the orders of the will.

For example, boxers are all "keyed up." Some of them have been spoken of as possessing "educated hands." The boxer proves that the hand is quicker than the eye. The fact that he is able to strike his opponent before his opponent is able to protect himself shows that at that instant his muscles possess greater irritability than do those of his adversary.

People who live in cold climates are much quicker in movement than those living in the tropics. I have found from my own experience that I possess more energy and more rapidity of motion when in the North than I do when in the South.

Interesting experiments may be had in gathering together a group of men of all types and classes. Have them stand in an exact line and just far enough away from a wall to enable them to reach it by simply extending the arm without moving the body. Have an electric current attached to each of them, worked by one switch, and then tell them to touch the wall as quickly as possible the instant they feel the current. You will find upon close observation that very few will touch the wall at the same time, and that the most responsive will touch it a second or more before the slowest or least responsive.

In our every-day walks of life we meet individuals who appear to us to be stupid; their actions are painfully slow. But in most cases the fault is not their own. They simply lack the irritability of muscle, and the quickness of nerve stimulus to the muscles from their brain which would enable them to produce rapid movements.

Although neither exercises of speed nor strength are necessary for the development of endurance, nevertheless they are essential for well-rounded fitness and physical preparedness; and experience in each will help greatly in anyone's endurance tests. There are many forms of endurance work which combine speed as well as strength, and the man who possesses wonderful endurance qualities alone would be helpless in the case of an emergency that required muscular strength as well. How many times have you read in the newspapers of someone jumping into the river to attempt to save the lives of one or more people who had overturned in a canoe some distance from the shore, only to lose his own life in his heroic endeavors? In nine cases out of ten the drowning person is so frightened that he wraps both arms and legs around his would-be rescuer in such grips that only a strong man can break them; and sometimes even the strong man cannot break them without the specific knowledge of how to break the holds of a panicky, drowning person. Therefore, I feel that a few words pertaining to strength work would prove just as interesting and just as valuable as anything I might write directly about endurance.

Whether the student indulges in weight lifting or in lifting the weight of his own body, it has the same effects upon his muscular system. I prefer the actual handling of my own body weight, for then not only is coordination of muscles exercised, but balance accomplishment and muscle sense, combined with the self-confidence obtained from the actual lifting of one's own weight, are developed. Let it not be understood that I shall endeavor to discuss body building or how to acquire great strength or development. These I have covered in my other books. But for actual value in the performance of endurance duties I much prefer the handling of my own weight to that of artificial weights, and would impress upon you the value of such exercises. In other words, I would rather perform ring and parallel or horizontal bar work for obtaining body coordination and increasing my endurance than I would artificial weight lifting.

Of course, a knowledge of each is essential to obtaining strength. You can chin and dip so many times a day, do what stunts you care to on the horizontal or parallel bars or on rings, and although you would in time possess a wonderful development, yet you would not be as strong nor have as bulging muscles as would an experienced weight lifter. On the other hand, if you confine your physical activities exclusively to heavy bar-bells and dumb-bells, you will make a very poor showing in endurance work, for you will be trained for short but powerful efforts.

I do not believe in sticking exclusively to one form of training. The work should be varied. For example, a person should exercise for a few minutes with an exerciser, then change for a few minutes to heavy dumb-bells—providing, of course, his body has been thoroughly trained and is in condition to use them. After a while the work should be changed to other forms. In this way only is it possible to produce the best possible all-round development, strength and endurance.

If you stick exclusively to one form of exercise year in and year out you will be like the day laborer who digs in the streets, who, although he may excel in his labor and is much better than you or I in that one thing, is absolutely useless in any other physical encounter or exertion that can be performed by the physical culture enthusiast. The topnotch boxer always will indulge in a little wrestling, handball and other pastimes besides his boxing. Of course, he will not do as much wrestling, for example, as boxing; his wrestling program, likely, would be limited to about one-twentieth of his boxing program. George Hackenschmidt, while a world's champion wrestler, also lifted weights, ran, jumped, tumbled, etc.

One form of exercise always helps one in doing another, and unless you intend to specialize in one certain sport, such as long distance running or swimming, I most heartily recommend exercise in all its varieties. Even though you care to specialize in just one thing, still it would do you no harm to have practical knowledge of all others, if they do not interfere with your specialization.

Gymnastic exercises, of course, rarely are feats of strength, and a well-accomplished gymnast oftentimes would make a poor showing in strength work. There are, however, movements performed with the aid of apparatus which at first seem to require an enormous expenditure of force, owing to the unfavorable positions in which the body levers act. But muscular effort in these movements is in direct ratio to the experience of the gymnast. By practice we become perfect, and on our road to perfection in our own line we make discoveries as we go along. Some seemingly difficult stunts easily could be performed! by the average athlete if he knew how. Often a slight variation or the learning of the required specific "knack" totally changes the conditions of the work. Therefore, an exercise which in the beginning seems hard to do, after a little practice becomes quite easy.

Wrestlers more closely come under the classification of strength workers than do gymnasts. Although wrestling does not consist of lifting weights, as usually considered, still the body weight of the opponent plus the opponent's resistance give the wrestler as much strength for his specific work as the weight lifter possesses for his. Undoubtedly, wrestling is the best all-round form of exercise in which one can indulge. There is hardly a part of the body that is not used, and, of course, certain parts receive more work than others. The neck, for example, obtains so much work that wrestlers as a rule possess necks that by many are considered over-developed. I have seen lightweight wrestlers, whose body weight was not more than one hundred and thirty-five pounds or one hundred and forty pounds and who did not stand more than five feet three or four inches in height, with necks measuring seventeen inches. A man of that height with such a neck may well be considered to be out of proportion. If he were five feet eight inches or taller a seventeen-inch neck would be in proportion to the rest of his body. Some of the champion heavyweight wrestlers have necks twenty-one and twenty-two inches in circumference, and yet these are in proportion because of the enormous bulk of these giants of strength. However, no matter how powerful a wrestler may be, nor how proficient in the science of wrestling, he would make a poor showing in gymnastics and other forms of endurance work if he did not indulge in them from time to time.

Exercises of strength demand the simultaneous action of a great number of muscles. They demand, further, that every muscle in action should bring its whole force into play. For this it is essential that the muscles have a very firm attachment to their fixed points on the bones. In other words, the ligaments and tendons must be exceedingly strong.

It is impossible for anyone to utilize his entire strength without producing a violent contraction of all the muscles of the trunk, the effect of which is to render the ribs motionless. That is why breathing must be suspended under a violent exertion. Next time you see anyone endeavoring to lift a very heavy object from the ground, observe the stiffening of the body from head to foot, and all the bones pressed together, so to speak, from the action of the muscles. Even the veins in the neck will stand out, and a redness will show in the face. He takes a deep breath and puts every muscle of his body, from his neck to his feet, into play. His entire body seems to go into rigid state; even the muscles of his face are violently contracted. In no other way can feats of strength be performed than by the coordination of the entire body. I once read of a strong man at a circus who could hold out heavy weights at arms' length with a smile upon his lips. He did it all right, but the smile was merely a grin in which the eyebrows and eyelids took no part. When you indulge in any great effort it is bound to make its showing upon the face, as the face muscles reflect the condition of the general musculature.

Exercises of strength cause less disturbance in the nervous system than do exercises of speed, and they do not demand, as do exercises of skill, any great brain work. The energetic and sustained muscular contractions draw the blood to the muscles in great quantity and keep it there for some time after the contractions. The muscular fibres benefit from this and increase in size. The blood is enriched with great quantities of oxygen, for increased respiratory need is the first effect of a great expenditure of muscular force. The blood, therefore, freely and easily circulates and satisfies the body's requirements in the period of repose which must follow each violent effort. The abdominal muscles contract during the deep breathing and produce a sort of massage upon the intestines. Nervous energy is held in reserve, and this is valuable for the repair of losses sustained in the work. The appetite is increased. It readily can be seen, therefore, that strength work, which is none other than muscle-building work, is of more benefit, physiologically and anatomically, than any other form of exercise. The heavy work tends to increase the weight of the individual, providing, of course, he does not carry around superfluous flesh at the start, in which case it would help to bring about reduction of weight.

It is possible for strength work to prove harmful to the beginner; and, having this in mind, I always have advocated that the student first of all build up his body with muscle-building exercise and strengthen his ligaments from this same work before attempting anything in the class of strength work. Rupture, dislocations, bursting of blood vessels, and even heart rupture are liable to occur during extra strains if the internal organs are not perfectly sound and strengthened by graduated exercise. Exhaustion, also, may result from work which exceeds one's strength, even though one receives the proper nourishment throughout.

If you wish to get from your muscles a quantity of force out of proportion to their contractile power, you will be obliged to make an energetic effort of will, and you will need a great amount of nervous energy to excite more powerfully your muscle fibres. In this case you will be performing work beyond your muscular strength, and will be working on nervous energy, and in time you will experience decrease in the size of your muscles, loss of general weight, and nervous exhaustion. Therefore, care should be taken in mapping out your strength-working program. You should not exercise beyond the point of fatigue in performing strength movements, any more than you should in performing speed movements or endurance work.

I believe everyone should devote at least five or ten minutes each day to lifting the weight of his body or else to the lifting of actual weights. Of course, when I say this I take it for granted that he has had enough preliminary training to put his muscles in condition to withstand this heavier exertion. It was only the other day that I jokingly asked a stout man how many times he could chin himself. He said about one-half a time, and to judge by the overweight he carried around with him, I think he was correct. Suppose this man were in a hotel fire, and he was forced by the smoke in his room to the window, from which he could see the lower part of the building in flames, and on the floor above a fireman was lowering a knotted rope which was tied securely in the room above. How do you suppose this fat man, to save his own life, could pull himself up hand over hand to the floor above when he did not have the ability to chin himself once, to say nothing of the twelve or fifteen times necessary to climb from one story to the next above?

Many times and in various ways the possession of strength may prove valuable in our lives. Ajax Whitman, a New York policeman who died recently, became famous years ago when he saved a little girl who was run over by a trolley car while playing in the street. Her body had become wedged between the wheels in such a way that it was impossible to get her out without moving the car. While waiting for the wrecking crew to make its appearance, this mighty policeman placed his back to the car, grasping a part securely with both hands behind his hips, bent his knees, and lifted the corner of the car high enough from the tracks for other rescuers to extricate the young one. Her life was saved.

The late Eugen Sandow, while out motoring not long ago, had an accident. The car was ditched and turned over. He escaped, but some of his friends were pinned underneath the car. This famous strong man lifted the automobile high enough that his friends could be released. It was this violent exertion in his fifty-seventh year that ruptured a blood vessel, from the effects of which he died late in 1925.

Though your strength may not play a part in some rescue of your own life from critical danger, it may in the lives of others; and if you who read this ever should have the opportunity of saving a life by your own physical endeavors, you will be amply repaid for all the efforts you have spent in the development of strength through the performance of strength work in addition to all the work you are doing strictly for the development of endurance.

One who, in order to adhere to the conventions of modern society, is afraid of obtaining calluses on the hands, or one who apparently is afraid of having his chest too deep or his shoulders too broad, will be just as helpless in a time of danger as was Yousef Mahmout, the giant Turkish wrestler of a generation ago, who sank with the ship while returning to his native land because he thought more of the gold in his belt, which he had around his waist and which made him sink, than he did of his own life. As this book is written for the purpose of teaching everyone to save his own life, it makes me reproachful of those who are afraid of a little additional muscular exertion; but the fact that you have read thus far shows that you are interested.

XI

EXERCISES of endurance are those in which the work must be continued for a considerable length of time. In these exercises the total expenditure of force is determined more by the duration than by the intensity or resistance, and rapidity of succession of the efforts. It is essential that the muscular effort should not be too great and the movements not too rapid, otherwise fatigue in some of its various forms may interrupt the movements too soon.

An exercise of endurance is only a moderate exercise if performed for a short time, but it may become forced exercise if it is continued too long. In these exercises the amount of work accomplished after a long time, even at the end of the day, for instance, may be very great; but the expenditure of force is made in such small fractions that there is no painful muscular effort at any movement; neither is there any marked disturbance in the functions of involved organs.

However, you may be able, in performing an exercise of endurance, to work up to the point, without knowing it, of making the exercise equivalent to heavy muscular work. When the limit of your own natural capacity is not exceeded, there is no noticeable disturbance created in the body. For the reason that in endurance work there is perfect balance between the muscular exertion and the power of resistance, you are able to go on working for a long time, allowing the useful effects of your exercising to accumulate, without causing any disturbance to the various organs or to the muscles used in the performance.

It is my opinion that a movement may be classed under endurance work even though it takes but fifteen or twenty minutes to reach the point of fatigue, and a light movement may be considered endurance work if it can be kept up for hours at a time. The two really blend and, of course, depend upon the strength and ability of the athlete. I consider that the one who chins himself forty to fifty times without stopping performs just as distinct an endurance movement as does the one who runs or swims a mile without resting.

Again, the object of this book is to enable everyone to save his own life; and I contend that heavy endurance work will prove just as valuable in this regard as will light endurance movements. If you are capable of climbing hand over hand up a long rope, say for one hundred feet, you can rest assured such a stunt and test of your muscles will be just as valuable to you as if you were able to swim one mile or to run two or three miles. Of course, if it is a specialty that you are interested in, such as becoming a long distance swimmer or a long distance runner or a twenty-five-round boxer, then whether you are able to chin yourself fifteen times or fifty times will make but little difference.

It is not my object to instruct anyone in any special line, nor to select any line of activity for anyone. If your ambition is to become a long distance runner you easily can obtain instructions and advice elsewhere. But, if, for example, you are unable to run more than fifty or one hundred yards without becoming fatigued and breathless, then the information I am endeavoring to impart, and the condition I am trying to interest you to acquire through this medium will prove valuable.

Have you ever noticed an athlete warming up just before a decisive event? This is noticed especially in track work; but if you have been observant in the gymnasium also, you may have noticed some prominent strong man going through a series of light calisthenic movements just before attempting heavier work. He is consciously getting his muscles supple and in condition for the necessary heavier exertions. This also can be done without direct intentional effort, as in long distance running when in endeavoring to cut down the time of the run one takes a trifle longer strides or runs with greater rapidity. The thought of winning acts as a stimulus and increases the speed and stride without any direct forced action of the will on the part of the athlete.

A person whose body is run down and weakened from lack of use, or a person who is recovering from a sickness will be greatly benefitted by endurance work. It is like giving food in fractional amounts to a convalescent. If upon recovering from a serious illness you were to eat a hearty meal, serious complications might arise, for when the digestion has been weakened and the requirements lessened by disease the food must be resumed in exceedingly small amounts and the amount increased very slowly. To give a weak person the amount of exercise at one period (if he were capable of doing it) that he would be doing after faithfully following athletic activities for many months would be fatal; but to start him with light endurance work of slow rhythm would enable him to receive the same value from the lighter exercise that the strong man receives from his heavy weights. In other words, the light endurance work to the feeble man is of just as much benefit as lifting heavy dumb-bells is to the weight lifter.

Therefore, the larger your muscles become and the stronger you become, the harder you must work in order to progress. A physical culturist usually has no difficulty in obtaining from a fourteen-inch to a sixteen-inch upper arm, depending, of course, upon his height; but it would be a most difficult matter for him to add another inch to this arm after he has been exercising for a year or two. The beginner, in performing one-tenth or less of the work done by the experienced athlete, derives just as much benefit, so far as girth increase and functional benefits are concerned, from his light endurance exercises as the experienced man receives from his greater work. Of course, as he becomes stronger he would get nowhere were he to continue with the same light endurance exercises. As he becomes stronger, organically and muscularly, he must progress accordingly in his type or degree of exercise or in both.

Endurance work must be divided into fractional quantities sufficiently small to enable the body to support each exercise dose without disturbing its normal functions. Also, the muscular efforts must be at sufficiently long intervals that the effect of the second effort may not be added directly to that of the first. Stated differently, there must be a long enough pause between each two movements to give the muscles and general energy a chance to recuperate. If there is not, the work instead of being endurance work, becomes muscle-building and, perhaps, in feeble cases, forced exercising.

As I have mentioned previously, the best example of endurance and of relaxation is the heart. It pumps all through life, but between beats there is enough pause to enable the heart muscle to recover. When the heart is overworked by being required to pump faster and harder than under normal conditions, it has insufficient time in which to rest between beats. Through such over-exertion the athlete gets what is called "athletic heart," and sometimes one or more leaking valves.

In an exercise of strength there is an accumulation of work, because each muscular effort is very evident, and one follows another before the full effect of the preceding has been entirely overcome. In an exercise of speed there is a multiplication of work, because of the rapid succession of efforts of small intensity. This leads in the end to an accumulation of work. In exercises of endurance the efforts, being repeated at sufficiently spaced intervals, are fractional, if at any time the amount of work performed does not exceed the power of resistance—though the final result is an accumulation of work, also.

An exercise of endurance is characterized by the necessity for perfect balance between the force of the muscular effort and the power of resistance in the body. It is difficult to determine just when an exercise is one of endurance when the work is not carried on in competition and does not become prolonged owing to destination—as in running, walking, swimming, etc. The same exercise may be classed in turn endurance, speed or strength exercise, according to the conditions under which it is performed. For instance, if you row in competition the work becomes speed work; whereas, if you row over a long course, mile after mile, it becomes endurance work. Rowing in very heavy seas takes on the form of strength work, just as walking, which is a type of endurance exercise, becomes strength work when you walk up-stairs or up-hill.

In other words, if you bring on fatigue too rapidly, it may be muscle-building, speed, or strength work and not endurance work; but if fatigue does not manifest itself and the work can go on continuously for long periods of time, it then is endurance work. Thus it is the conditions under which you perform the exercise that determine its character.

But individual conditions, of training, strength, wind, and nervous energy, have much to do with determining the type of exercise, also. There is nothing so variable as the power of resistance within different people. What is an exercise of strength or speed for one becomes endurance for another who has had much exercising experience. Taking rowing again for illustration, this is an exercise of strength to the man who is learning, for in a short time he is out of breath; but to the experienced oarsman who spends much of his time on the water it becomes endurance work, for he can keep it up all day without fatiguing.

Generally, the difference in the power of resistance, or the staying power, as it also may be called, of different people is due largely to the difference in their respiratory powers. It might be said that one's respiratory fitness is the true regulator of all work of endurance. A person whose rib-box is narrow would not stand the same chance in competition as one whose rib-box is broad. In the former, the lungs are not as large, nor have they the room to expand

; whereas not only is the lung capacity greater in the one whose rib-box is wide but his endurance powers excel in direct proportion.

There are two conditions, then, necessary to form an exercise of endurance. The first is a certain moderation in the force of the exercises. The second is a certain power of resistance on the part of the body. Therefore, stamina or staying power applies rather to the qualities of a man than it concerns the nature of the work he performs. A work of endurance is one in which the method of performance enables one to continue it for a long time; and the man with staying power is one whose body is fit to support prolonged work. Some people are unable to perform the most moderate exercise without showing, after a very short time, the signs of extreme fatigue. There are others who keep up, with astonishing powers of resistance, the most violent work; and, as I said, for them the exercise of strength or speed becomes merely an exercise of endurance.

While at a summer resort one day I noticed from my window a man skipping a rope on a platform which had been placed on the sand. This rope skipping is done by every little girl in her early childhood days; and it also is indulged in by athletes, for it is very beneficial for the wind and the muscles below the knee. It was about ten o'clock in the morning when I first saw this man skipping the rope. I watched him for a few minutes and then went about my daily duties. Around noon-time I again saw him skipping the rope, and learned to my astonishment, upon investigation, that he had been skipping the rope continuously for those two hours. It was remarkable that he could do so practically without a miss, and still more remarkable that his lungs and heart were in such a phenomenal condition as to function properly while withstanding the obvious and necessary exertion. Jumping off the ground, no matter how lightly it is done, affects the heart and respiratory organs considerably, and it must have taken much practice for this man to be able to continue this one form of exercise for so long a time. I know I shouldn't have the patience to do it. However, it surely was a marvelous display of endurance.

But place a rope in the hands of the beginner and ask him to skip for five minutes; and, even though he possess the technique and can perform without a miss, he will find that his exertions will bring on breathlessness with such rapidity and tiring of the muscles of his calves and shins so quickly that to him the work, for the short time it would be possible, would be muscle-building.

Rope skipping is an excellent exercise for creating endurance, both in the muscles below the knee and in your staying power or wind. For the beginner, rope skipping may prove a violent exercise; but after practice and to the experienced physical culturist it becomes endurance work. If after an exercise you experience neither fatigue nor breathlessness, you have been performing endurance movements, and you may consider yourself fit for that work. If, instead, you are winded and any part of your body is tired, you have been performing violent exertions. This is one way to distinguish violent exercising from endurance work or gentle exercise—for endurance consists of taking exercise as easily as possible. By continuing the movement for a longer time than usual, fatigue and breathlessness will occur in endurance work; but it will come on more slowly and gradually than in the performance of violent exercise.

In order that you may perform an exercise that may be continued for a long time, the first condition is that it does not lead to breathlessness. You can go on walking, for example, in spite of weary legs and sore feet; but you cannot go on running when you are out of breath. Certain parts of the body naturally possess more endurance than others. This, of course, becomes localized. For instance, the fingers and hands naturally have more endurance than have the shoulders or the back. We are continually using the fingers and hands in our everyday life; therefore, they seem almost wholly immune to fatigue. Observing the pianist at the motion picture theatre who continues playing throughout the various continuous performances, you often wonder why he does not become exhausted. True, he has periods of relaxation; but his fingers are capable of continuing their light endurance efforts much longer than would the muscles of his arms and shoulders.

The muscles around the jaw seem to possess tireless endurance qualities, especially in those whom we often observe who are continually chewing gum. Not long ago there was a public speaker who continued talking, without a letup, for forty-eight hours, while I often have gotten tired after talking ten or fifteen minutes. My experience has taught me to say little and listen more, and I presume that is the reason I notice the effort of speaking more than do the public speakers and many others.

If you attempt any exercise or movement of endurance, it is essential that you eliminate all extra effort from the action. The absence of effort saves you from the violent exertion of the heart and blood vessels which hinders the working of these organs. The object of endurance exercise, therefore, is to spare the organs as much as possible, and it is most essential to give the body the chance to repair even during the work. In this way breathlessness will not occur during exercises of endurance. By such care the quantity of carbonic acid produced by the activity of the muscles never rises to a quantity in excess of that which the lungs can eliminate, but it is removed from the blood as fast as it is formed and passes unnoticed from the body. It is possible to escape breathlessness while performing endurance work only by introducing considerable oxygen into the body by way of the respiratory system.

Proper training, therefore, is the first step towards acquiring endurance. The object of training is to fit you as completely and as quickly as possible for the performance of a given work. In other words, it is preparation. Again, training has other meanings besides muscular activities. A diver may be trained in holding his breath longer. Jockies are trained to make them lighter so as to lighten the work of the horses that carry them. Hence, in order to continue being in the condition in which training puts you, it is necessary to keep up that training, in considerable degree, at least. Otherwise you simply go back to about where you were when you started.

It is well always to keep in good condition, though I do not believe in being "on edge," so to speak, at all times. By this I mean that if you were training for a contest, such as boxing, wrestling or running, it would be a waste of nervous force to continue day after day the condition that you should be in for the contest. If this condition is kept up one becomes stale, and staleness demands a rest.

Getting and keeping in good condition does not necessarily mean the loss of weight, unless, of course, superfluous flesh exists upon your body. Once you have eliminated excess fatty tissue, you will not lose weight by moderate training. You will further lose, however, if you are over training and, as I said before, continually keyed up to the highest pitch. An athlete who once becomes muscular, even though he were thin before he indulged in physical culture work, generally will accumulate fat if he discontinues his training and relaxes, just as the fat man who reduces to symmetrical proportions will quickly resume his old-time pudgy figure if he discontinues his exercise. Of course, there will be a falling off in the contour and size of the muscles, and fatty tissue will accumulate around the most inactive parts, such as the waistline and hips.

The thin individual reacts somewhat differently. He usually continues to take on more weight as his muscles increase in size, but should he stop training he not only would rapidly lose an inch or more from his thighs and arms, but he would increase an inch or more around his torso and especially around the waist.

I tried an experiment myself a few years ago on the effect of prolonged relaxation. As you know, I am an advocate of daily exercise, and I practice what I preach; but for an experiment on this occasion I suddenly dropped off training and did nothing for three weeks. Now my waist measured thirty inches before ending my training; but upon the completion of the three weeks' rest it measured thirtysix, and I had the devil's own time getting it back again to thirty-two inches, where it has remained, refusing to become any smaller; and, of course, I in turn refuse to allow it to become any larger. While in training my upper arm measured sixteen and one-half inches. After the three weeks of relaxation it measured fifteen and three-quarter inches. My thigh measured twenty-three and one-half inches, and after my lay-off, strange to say, it increased to twenty-four inches. The girth of my chest gained one inch during my period of inactivity.

During this period of rest I was not my normal self organically and mentally. I felt sluggish and lost considerable physical ambition, and it was very hard to start into exercising again. This is the only time I have experimented in this way, and I can assure you that I have no desire to do it again; for I have found that there is nothing equal to keeping fit at all times and in such a condition that it requires but a day or two of extra training to fit you for any contest.

Professional boxing offers an interesting example of training methods. Usually it takes about six weeks of preparation for a fighter to fit himself for a contest, and upon the evening of the contest his muscles and nerves are keyed up to the highest point of responsiveness. If after the bout he were asked to continue his active training, he soon would find himself stale, both mentally and physically—mentally, perhaps, because there would be no incentive for him to keep it up, and physically, because of the drain upon his body. Fighters, you know, perform considerable endurance work and often spend from two to three hours a day at their work-out. If this were kept up continually it soon would wear them out. Therefore, relaxation after a contest is necessary, and in most cases fighters add considerable weight during their periods of inactivity.

I believe in carrying from three to five pounds of extra weight on my body at all times, as it gives me something to work off—something to feed on, so to speak. If a boxer continued his daily endurance training right up to the day of the contest, he would be apt to find himself stale during the encounter. That is why fighters usually relax on the day the bout is to take place. This gives the muscles the relaxation necessary before their final exertion. It would be well for anyone who trains for a contest, whether it be boxing, wrestling, rowing, running or what not, to follow the fighter's program by relaxing and avoiding all physical activities on the day of the event. The object of training is to develop your muscular and nervous energy and to increase your power of resisting fatigue. If you have not secured these effects by training before the last day it is occur frequently and regularly at all times; the muscles quite certain that you cannot develop it on the last day.

As I have mentioned so many times, relaxation should should be given brief periods of rest after each movement in order to recuperate properly for another exertion. How would you expect to run a mile or more if you ran the first hundred yards at top speed? And how would you expect to box twenty rounds if at the sound of the gong in the opening round you exerted yourself by boxing at top speed? You may be able to go at top speed during part of any contest; but the time for this is well along in the contest after slower work allowing some degree of relaxtion, which permits the vital organs and muscles to reach their highest degree of harmonious action.

In violent exercising, fatigue and breathlessness come on quite suddenly, yet they leave you more quickly than do the fatigue and breathlessness produced by the performance of endurance work. I have seen swimmers come out of the water, after swimming a couple of miles, and although they were breathing somewhat above normal they were not as winded as sprinters I have seen who have gone but one hundred yards through the waters. As a rule, sprinting swimmers upon completion of their destination are quite winded, yet after a short period of rest they would be able to make another sprint. But an endurance swimmer would not have any inclination to get into the water soon for another long swim after the completion of one endurance test. This is because his fatigue has come on gradually, and is more general and more lasting than the fatigue of the sprinter. You can experience these reactions yourself; and, after all, you will find experience the best teacher.

I have watched the performances of Joe and Adolph Nordquest, the two brothers from Ashtabula, Ohio, who are noted for their strength performances. I have had the pleasure of seeing Joe put up with the left hand overhead, three hundred and one pounds, creating a new world's record for the left arm bent press. It was interesting to note how he walked around the long bar-bell about a dozen times before he attempted to touch it. He was working himself up to a physical and mental pitch in order to successfully perform the lift. After raising the bell overhead with one arm and dropping it to the floor the exhalation of his breath sounded like a bellows, so forcibly did it come out of his lungs. He was quite winded from the exertion; yet after only a minute or two he was fully capable of attempting other lifts.

I watched his brother Adolph lift a huge bar-bell, two hands overhead, about ten or twelve times. This was done in a public performance, and the weight was announced as two hundred and fifty pounds. Knowing him personally, I inquisitively asked him, after the performance, what the actual weight of the bell was. Adolph in a whisper confided to me, at the same time asking me not to tell anyone, that the weight actually was only two hundred and fortyfive pounds. It doesn't seem very much to relate or to read; but anyone who cares to attempt to lift even a two hundredpound bar-bell over his head ten times will appreciate the marvelous strength Adolph Nordquest possesses. But I am rambling from my subject. After completing the lifts his part in the performance was ended and he was quite winded; but I am sure he could have duplicated the whole thing after a minute or two of relaxation.

It will be of interest and value for you to have a little knowledge of the effects of exercises of strength. All exercises are in the same category. Strength work really blends with endurance work; because, as I have stated previously, what is endurance work for one is strength work for another. To the beginner, the lifting of a fifty-pound dumbbell from the floor to arms' length overhead would mean performing a feat of strength, while an athlete who did this movement before me three hundred and fifty times without stopping really performed an endurance test.

As related previously, I give a great many of my pupils in their first lesson the common push-up or floor dip exercise. This is quite a stunt for some of them to do, especially if they have never exercised before. But if I were to give this exercise to those who have had six or eight months or more of training they would consider it as simply a warming-up movement. I feel that everyone should perform strength work and continue with the strength movements until they become endurance repetitions. There is really no distinct line of separation between strength work and endurance work. They blend into each other; and it depends wholly on the individual whether the exercise or movement undertaken is one of strength or one of endurance.

The state of mind is an important factor in the performance of endurance work. During all training for endurance work your mind must be free from all mental disturbances and all depressing emotions. You must avoid all nervous excitement and all keen sensations, and, as I have previously stated, peace and harmony should prevail. One who trains for endurance should not perform any violent exercise. Violent exercise need not necessarily mean a feat of strength or a different stunt; it may be any violent exertions that would bring on fatigue too rapidly; and fatigue should be avoided in training for endurance.

In the performance of heavy work, which may be classed as strength exercising, there are two important factors necessary—the straining of the muscles and the forcing of your will power. It is important, therefore, that you understand the value of nervous energy throughout these performances, as it plays a more important part than you may think.

I recall the great English weight lifter, Edward Aston, whose weight is around one hundred and sixty pounds; yet he has successfully lifted, one arm overhead, three hundred and one pounds in the bent press. I also recall the last time I met Anton Matysek, the phenomenal lifter of Baltimore, whose weight at the time was about one hundred and sixtyfive pounds and yet he successfully lifted almost three hundred pounds in the bent press method, one hand overhead; and his other feats with the dumb-bells also have been remarkable. Each of these men weighed less than I do and a great many of their muscles are smaller in measurement than mine; and yet they are capable of lifting considerably more poundage than I have ever been able to lift. For me to bent press two hundred or two hundred and twentyfive pounds was quite a feat of strength; but to lift the same weight would have been merely play for Aston or Matysek. Undoubtedly, they possessed more nervous energy than I did when lifting the weights, and, of course, they have had considerable more practice with dumb-bells and bar-bells than I have had, for I very seldom use them. If I had practiced as faithfully with the weights as they had, perhaps

I might have been in the same class with them; yet, I may not have been.

Variations in nervous energy may be manifested in a physical manner by a more or less evident stimulation of the muscles, which produces more or less powerful muscular contractions. Doubtless, this difference in nervous energy largely explains why two men of the same size and weight differ greatly in their feats of strength. But the exertion of a weight lifter endeavoring to lift an enormous weight from the ground overhead with two arms is no greater in proportion to strength possessed than it would be for the beginner to lift light weights or to chin himself for the first time.

To one who is accustomed to lifting weights it is an easy matter to pull himself up a rope hand over hand. While lifting weights may constitute violent exercises and feats of strength, it produces such strength that it makes rope climbing a mere test of endurance for the muscles involved. To one who is accustomed to curling a heavy bar-bell it is an easy matter to perform a great number of chins on a horizontal bar. Such rope climbing and chinning should be indulged in by everyone, for it may prove necessary sometime for saving your own life, though I hope not. The beginner who cannot chin himself once or dip between parallel bars more than two or three times is really in a regretable state regarding his personal safety in the event of some dangers. The mere act of chinning himself once or dipping once or twice is, to him, really a feat of strength. Therefore, he should continue at such strength work until he is able to perform a number of repetitions, and after the repetitions become prolonged the work can be classed as endurance movements.

If an experienced athlete for the first time were to take a spade and dig a deep hole in the ground he would be performing strength movements, even though such labor would be endurance work for the working man. The athlete, whose muscles are used in certain ways and who is accustomed to fifteen or twenty minutes of exercising daily, would be working his muscles in a different manner in throwing over his shoulder spadefuls of dirt, and he would soon tire, just as the experienced weight lifter, who is used to lifting enormous weights, would become tired very quickly while wielding the axe for chopping down a tree.

It depends upon how the muscles are used whether the work is a movement of strength or a movement of endurance. The lumberjack who can swing the axe in cutting down tree after tree without fatigue and with scarcely a show of perspiration on his forehead, undoubtedly would make a poor showing at lifting dumb-bells or in running at top speed for any short distance. Also, he most likely would find himself breathless were he to cross-country trot for a mile or more. On the other hand, the sprinter or the crosscountry runner soon would tire wielding the axe.

Therefore, strength movements and endurance movements are so closely associated that their type can be determined only by the condition and ability of the person performing them. Thus it can be seen that it is best for everyone to indulge in all forms of exercise, light and heavy; for the light work always can be accomplished with practice and with the development of the wind, while the heavy strength movements will develop into those of endurance, which light exercises cannot do.

XII

IT IS INTERESTING to note the general effects produced by similar exercises upon different individuals. When you enter the gymnasium for the first time you see the stout man going through the same movements as his thin neighbor. You may wonder if these movements that the stout individual is performing will be of any benefit to the thin fellow; yet, if you were to return to the gymnasium after an absence of a few months and if these same individuals had continued to work daily, you would find that the stout one had lost weight while the thin one had gained weight. This is because exercising produces two different effects. In the thin person it increases the bodily tissue while in the stout person it decreases the fatty tissue. These apparently different effects may be summed up in one chief effect, however, and that it is the development of more nearly normal metabolism or tissue processes.

There are a certain number of muscles in the human body, and a stout person has practically the same muscular tissue as a thin person of the same general type and original build. You cannot see them developed in the fat man owing to his covering of fat, but you can plainly discern them in the developed thin individual because they stand out owing to lack of fatty tissue on them. The fat man most likely will have somewhat larger (though perhaps softer) muscles hidden under his fat than has the thin man. This is because he weighs more and naturally has to carry around a greater weight than the thin one, thus giving his muscles more exercise; his muscles should be larger in proportion to the amount of work they do. But when both the thin man and the fat man, after a sufficient period of training, reach more nearly the point of bodily perfection their muscles will be very little different in size, though they may be considerably different in contour.

From this we can see that the need for exercise is felt just as much by thin people who assimilate too little as by fat people who assimilate too much. The need for exercise, then, depends upon one of two physiological necessities, the intensity of which gives us warning. It comes from an overcharge with reserve materials, and the urgent necessity that these materials should be burned; or it may arise from a general sluggishness of the functions and the need of a stimulus capable of arousing them to a fresh activity.

By this time you will realize the value of being in condition and keeping the muscles fit, for one who has any weak part in his make-up cannot expect to qualify in any test of endurance.

I must admit that my greatest interest is in body building, and I sometimes find it difficult to refrain from branching off to that subject. But as I have covered this is another book I will only touch upon the high spots in your physical make-up.

Let us consider the neck. A strong neck will prove valuable in many instances, but would be of little use in any endurance work. Nevertheless, the trapezius muscles, which run well up into the rear of the neck, are used in most movements of the shoulders and arms, in addition to strictly neck movements. Therefore, the neck will receive considerable work in a great number of endurance exercises. Rowing and swimming, for instance, bring into play to a great extent the trapezius muscles.

The forearm and upper arm muscles must be fit, for they will be used in all climbing exertions.

The value of strong legs need hardly be emphasized. When the muscles of the thighs and calves coordinate properly they not only will pull you through many an emergency, but through the development of a good pair of legs you can be assured of good respiratory power. As I have mentioned, it is impossible to perform vigorous leg movements without calling heavily upon the lungs.

As important as the muscles are in performing endurance work, I consider the lungs of greater importance, for it is in the respiratory organs that the first sign of fatigue is felt. The amount of air entering the lungs is regulated by the capacity of the lungs, and, of course, by the demand for air, by exercises or work. Therefore, it is of great importance that the muscular work you do is such as to increase the size of the cavity in which the lungs are contained and the lungs themselves.

So many people, and I can truthfully say the majority of people, breathe with but a small part of their lungs. Singers and wind-instrument musicians are in a class by themselves when it comes to lung capacity. Their excellent chest cavities are developed unconsciously through their chest and lung exercises incident to their professions. However, the average individual can obtain just as remarkable a lung capacity as any singer or musician who plays the cornet, trombone or other wind instrument, by practicing forced breathing.

The amateur physical culturist lays too little stress upon the importance of deep breathing, and considers the simple arm movements which throw the shoulders back sufficient to increase his lung capacity and the size of his rib-box. But he is sadly in error. Accumulation of work is really the only way to obtain   good   lungs and staying power.   By accumulation of work I mean the combined performance of exercises of strength, speed and endurance. Where the arms alone perform the work you will find very little breathlessness occurring; but where the arms unite with the legs in performing exercises you will find yourself quickly becoming winded.

Leg exercise requires much more work than that which is performed by the arms. The muscles of the upper limbs could not support without extreme fatigue an expenditure of force that could be borne by the lower limbs with small effort. It is an easy matter to walk a mile; but where is there a gymnast or a strong man who could walk a mile along a horizontal rod or ladder while hanging from his hands? The total mechanical work, however, would be the same, displacing the same weight through the same horizontal distance.

When fatigue overtakes you and you are breathless, the act of satisfying your thirst for air naturally will be of wonderful benefit to the lungs, yet it will not expand the chest nor increase its size as much as forced deep breathing under normal conditions. As the legs possess practically three times the strength of the arms they are capable of producing three times the amount of work. But if the lungs are not in perfect working order, that is if the rib-box is not flexible and the lung capacity not great enough, the same performance of leg work will exhaust you in a shorter time than would arm exercise, even though, as I said, the legs are much stronger than the arms. Consideration must be taken of the weight of the body which the legs must carry; and, naturally, greater effort constantly is brought upon them than upon the arms.

A great many teachers of exercise are in error regarding the development of lung power, as so many of them advocate the simple raising of the arms to raise the rib-box and thereby increase the depth of the chest and lung cavity. Such exercise may be good for loosening the rib-box, and perhaps when accompanied by deep inhalations will add an inch or two to the chest; but, as I stated before, real lung power can be developed only by actual endurance practice. Walking along the street and taking one hundred deep inhalations a day, for example, will not benefit you to any great extent in the development of endurance. The best exercise for increasing the size of the chest is that which compels the deepest inhalations—natural inhalations, and not those consciously and intentionally produced by the will.

You can experiment along these lines yourself. You may swing your arms, bend your body from side to side, or perform all manner of twists and calisthenic movements, and yet breathlessness will not come on as quickly as it will by a short vigorous sprint, whether it be in running, swimming, rowing or the like. After such a sprint the lungs are fairly crying for more air, with the consequence that you will be compelled to inhale as much oxygen as possible in order to satisfy the craving.

One cannot expect to excel in any feat of endurance unless first of all he gives attention to his lung capacity and rib-box. All endurance work requires staying power— good wind. It is true that good lung capacity and wind will be developed from the practice of endurance work; but endurance work will come much easier if lung development is gotten before the endurance work begins. The finest-built athlete, whose arms may have reached the strong man's proportions and whose pectoral or breast muscles may stand out in pleasing contour, likely will possess a comparatively narrow chest in spite of his development if his lungs are weak.

I frequently attend a gymnasium and play handball with the instructor there. This man has practically no muscular development to speak of; but what an enormous chest he has! His rib-box is wide, and the deepest part of his chest seems to be below the breast bone, and when viewed from the side, when he stands erect and has his chest somewhat expanded, it takes on the appearance of a high, fleshy abdomen. This fellow finds no difficulty in playing twelve or fifteen games of handball without stopping. And though his muscles are of a different type entirely from those of the weight lifter or strong man, still they are more pliable and have considerably more endurance. His staying powers seem to be perfect, and all this I ascribe mainly to his wonderful lung capacity and the flexibility of his ribbox.

If you wish to develop the chest, do not try to do so by raising the ribs, but by trying to inflate all the air cells of the lungs. You cannot do this by any mechanical means; and the most voluntary muscular movements would not produce the results obtainable by forced aspirations.

The lungs are increased in size as a result of forced respirations which make them work better. Under the influence of unusual exercise the air cells increase in size and contain more air. Also, more blood is supplied to them. Their capillary network becomes more pronounced, and, in consequence, their nutrition is more active. Accordingly, they take up more room. It is in this manner that the regular working of the great number of air cells that ordinarily are inactive can rapidly increase the size of the lungs.

In order to increase the size of the chest and the lung capacity the work must begin from the inside, and not from the outside by the simple working of the muscles. Oxygen must be forced in, and as the lungs expand and become larger they press against the ribs, stretching the cartilages between the ribs and finally spreading the ribs farther apart. Exercise, it is true, can be of great assistance in increasing the quality of the lung tissue. For instance, if the arms are held overhead when taking deep inhalations, naturally the ribs are elevated and more in a position to receive the pressure of the lungs from the inside. You would not expect to take very deep breaths while sitting in a crouched position. It is only natural that you throw your shoulders back and raise the rib-box as much as possible while performing deep inhalations. Increasing the size of the chest, then, is done chiefly by the work of the lungs.

It is not a fair measurement to consider the size of the strong man's chest when passing the tape around the chest under the arm pits, because of his outstanding latissimus dorsi muscles, those beefy yet pleasingly proportioning hills of flesh that cause the slant from the arm pits to the waist line. The thickness of his pectoral, or breast muscles, also adds considerable to his chest measurement. Although many strong men show enormous chests, both in appearance and measurement, many of them possess weak lungs. If I were to have my choice and could accept only one or the other, I most certainly would select the body which has a big lung capacity rather than the large and muscular body containing weak lungs. With a good chest and lung capacity it is an easy matter to add muscular tissue in proportion. I at least would be assured that the amount of oxygen entering my lungs at each inhalation would purify my blood and keep me immune to sickness and disease and fill me with the robust health that everyone should experience.

If you have a good lung capacity to begin with, the practice of endurance movements will come much easier to you than if you endeavor to build up your lung capacity and rib-box by means of endurance exercises. Let us say that we have a thin man and a husky chap who start to exercise at the same time. Neither ever has worked physically before. After each has performed exactly the same exercises for a period of about six months, it will be found that the burly chap quite evidently has made better progress and will be much stronger than his thin competitor. This is because he had a good foundation to begin with. Hence, if you have a good flexible rib-box and a fine lung capacity you have every advantage in your favor when you begin training for endurance work.

Since the muscles play a most important part in endurance work it is essential that we look into the general effects of exercise upon them in order to learn more of their capabilities. Among the most striking effects of muscular exercise are the changes undergone by the muscles themselves under the influence of work. They lose much of the fat between their fibres, it being burned up by the activities; and by persistent daily efforts they gradually increase in size. But loss of fat and increase in size are not the only changes observed in the muscles as the result of work. You can notice also a change in shape, depending upon the movement the muscle performs. This is one of the most interesting of the local effects of work.

A muscle which is more constantly in action than other muscles, or in other words a muscle which contracts more often than its antagonist, undergoes in the end a certain degree of shortening. This is very noticeable in the arms of some indoor physical culture enthusiasts. I have observed young fellows who have exercised with five-pound dumbbells whose bicep muscle was so shortened that the lower part did not break or slant into the proper place on the upper forearm but seemed to be attached to the humerus or bone of the upper arm. This, of course, was not the case, as all biceps are attached to the radius bone of the forearm. The movement this one man in particular had performed consisted of curling the five-pound dumb-bells from the arms hanging at his sides so that the bells touched his shoulders alternatelyduring the curling movements. Evidently he had been lowering the bells but not fully straightening the arms. Hence, there was always a tension upon the belly of the biceps, which in turn became shortened and naturally lacked the power that it would have had if the break or downward slant of its lower extremity had gone into the proper place. Such a development might be called a deformity of the muscle.

This same thing can occur in any muscle or group of muscles in the body. That is, they can be worked or exercised improperly, with the result that they not only will lack the contour they could have if exercised properly but they will lack the strength, also.

You may wonder how the shape of the muscle could possibly affect endurance. But if the muscle is improperly developed and shortened this most assuredly will have some reducing effect upon the leverage and coordination essential in all endurance tests. Muscles for endurance must be long and pliable. Of course, they also can have bulk and size; but if the development through the exercise performed is merely bulk of muscle, it will require changing of routine and plans of training in order to qualify the muscles for endurance work. If, for example, you persist in training with heavy dumb-bells you naturally will acquire huge muscles, and they will be strong, as well; but in all probability they will be useless in performing endurance tests.

If you divide your exercises and mix them, so to speak— performing some strengthand muscle-building work and some endurance work—the muscles, while probably not reaching the measurements, bulk and contour that they would have reached if you had trained exclusively for development, yet would be far more useful to you; and you would be able to accomplish a great deal more whenever you felt like it, even though you lacked the halfinch or so of girth that you could have gotten by eliminating all light movements.

The desire to continue exercising lessens as one becomes older. This is simply a law of human nature, or appears to be. Frequently the one ambition of a young man in his teens is to become as big and strong as possible. He thinks only about a chest or upper arm measuring so many inches. If he can but develop certain Herculean proportions he feels that he will be absolutely satisfied with life and that there would not be another thing that he would wish for. But as he becomes a little older and realizes that robust health, sound heart and lungs and more endurance are of more concern and benefit to him than the more showy muscles and entertaining strength, he is more apt to discontinue his heavy training and adopt methods more suitable for his years and his more mature aims.

As a rule, when a man reaches thirty he is through with exercising; and most men in the thirties are pitifully out of shape, muscularly, bodily and functionally. It would be folly for anyone to continue vigorous training with heavy dumb-bells when he reaches the late thirties, and yet there are a few who keep it up. That is why we often read that "another strong man dies young." It is not only folly, but it is fatal to force oneself to continue year after year with the most strenuous exercise that one performed during his youth. If you are young and a weight-lifting enthusiast or an advocate of heavy exercise, bear in mind that much of the muscle tissue you have acquired from such work positively will be replaced by fat if, when you grow older, you discontinue your training.

The habit of exercise is an essential one to form for the development and preservation of best health; but no matter how well developed the habit may be, it will be against nature's law to continue well into middle life if the work is of very strenuous variety.

I repeat, if you persist in lifting the weights and performing heavy dumb-bell exercises and do not do any light endurance movements in conjunction with such training, your muscles will prove worthless in any endurance test, and so also will every organ concerned with such tests. If, on the other hand, you are interested in all endurance work and do not have that youthful desire for bulk or great strength, you would profit much more by adopting and continuing such methods of training as would develop endurance, for you would possess muscles and staying power that would last for many years longer, should you at any time become lax in your physical activities or entirely discontinue them.

To a swimmer who is capable of swimming a mile or more (and it is very easy to swim a mile after you have mastered the art of swimming) it would be a very easy matter to swim a quarter of a mile or more even though he had not entered the water for a period of many years. But a sprinter or short distance swimmer, who is used to one hundred or two hundred and twenty-yard sprints, would find himself all out of condition were he to attempt to swim his accustomed distance or even less, after he had absented himself from the water for a few years.

Take the runner for example, also. Even if one who had had the ability to trot along for a mile or two sat at a desk for several years and did no running at all, he still would find himself capable of running a fair distance; whereas another individual who never had run more than one hundred yards in his life, would find himself greatly fatigued from his exertions were he to attempt to run his accustomed distance after a few years lay-off.

From this it can be seen that prolonged movement or endurance work is of more value in later years than the violent exertions which give the muscles bulk and strength. These statements may seem questionable, but I suggest that you experiment for yourself and find out. If you have specialized in any one form of athletics, even though you have not done any athletic work in that line for a long time, you will find yourself more capable of performing or accomplishing movements in the line you excelled in than you would in any other form of physical activity. But this is particularly true if you have done endurance work of some kind.

I have known a certain insurance man in Brooklyn for a number of years, and many times have seen medals and cups which he won in his youth for high jumping. I think he is now in his fifties; but he possesses the body of a man in the thirties, although he has done practically no physical training at all for several years. A year or so ago, when crossing the street, an automobile was almost upon him before he saw it. With quick presence of mind—more, in reality, an instinctive muscular response—he jumped— not forward but upward, so that his legs straddled the hood of the car. Outside of a few minor bruises he ascaped uninjured. But the ability in high jumping that he still possessed undoubtedly saved his life. This also shows an interesting case of unconscious or instinctive muscular reaction or response. Had this man been a broad jumper he undoubtedly would have jumped forward; but because he had excelled in high jumping, the first thought flashed to the muscles of his legs propelled him upward.

The reader must not misunderstand me and think I am condemning strength and the means of its development. In one chapter I recommend strength work, and now it may seem that I am somewhat opposing it. But I am not. Muscles that are strong and capable of great exertions will prove just as useful in many cases of emergency as will muscles capable of endurance only; and I want to impress upon you the value of the power of physical self protection. What I am endeavoring to set forth is that muscles should possess endurance qualities just as much as or even more than bulk and strength. The two should be combined. If you combine endurance movements and strength movements you can obtain a harmonious and pleasing development even though you may not secure the maximum girth that you would if you remained exclusively with strength training. But is it not worth while to sacrifice half an inch, let us say, of girth to possess muscles that will prove capable, should the emergency arise, of saving your life or that of another?

If you exercise exclusively with heavy dumb-bells or barbells for purposes of developing strength and muscle bulk, you will obtain the maximum girth and the maximum strength that your frame work and capabilities permit and warrant. But in order to maintain the same bulk year after year you must continue such exertions and stick to progressive exercising. If you do not you will find your muscles decreasing in size half an inch or more. And yet, it will be impossible for you to continue the violent strengthbuilding exercises in later years that you are capable of performing in your youth. Your energies would not permit the continuance, and, as I have said before, if it were possible to continue, it would prove disastrous.

Suppose you performed dumb-bell exercise for a year or two and you developed a sixteen-inch upper arm, a forty-five-inch normal chest, and other parts of your body in proportion. In order to maintain the sixteen-inch arm and forty-five-inch chest you must continue using the same amount of resistance or weight; or, if you want to maintain your maximum measurements or become a little larger if possible, you must increase the resistance or weight. This can go on year after year, but as you leave your twenties and climb up in the thirties your vitality would not be as great as it was in your youth. Your enthusiasm likely would lessen, also; and to continue such vigorous training you would be forced to call upon your reserve powers, nervous energy, and will power. Your body would not recuperate as quickly from the effects of the exertion as it used to. And should you continue such heavy training methods the time would come some day when the weakest link of the chain would snap, and there would be said of you, "another strong man dies young."

Now let us suppose that you do not devote your entire time to dumb-bell exercise but divide your exercising period into about fifteen minutes of the heavy work and about fifteen or twenty minutes or more of light work. After a year or two, instead of having a sixteen-inch arm and a forty-five-inch chest, suppose you had a fifteen and a half-inch arm and a forty-four inch chest. The contour of your muscles would be just as pleasing even though they lacked this half inch in the arm and inch in the chest, and other parts accordingly. However, your muscles could outlast the muscles of the exclusive heavy weight lifter, and you would be able to accomplish things that would make the dumb-bell artist sit back with envy. As you grew older and entered your thirties you would still possess the fifteen and a half-inch arm and forty-four-inch chest, because these measurements were developed through more natural exertions and were not forced, as are the ones of the heavy weight enthusiast.

If at the older period of life, you were to discontinue endurance work and exercise exclusively with violent work for a shorter period of time than you would in your youth, you might easily increase the girth of your measurements for the time being. But here again, to continue such violent work would be unwise. Muscles developed by the use of heavy weights are never as pliable as those developed by endurance movements. You readily can see, then, that no matter how hard you may work physically in your youth and how much progress you may make with heavy weight exercises, you positively will lose some of the strength and some of the measurements and contour of your muscles as you become older. On the other hand, if you combine endurance movements with muscle- and strength-building movements, you will be more inclined to maintain for a much longer period the proportions that you have gotten from such methods of training, because the strain is not so great upon the organs, and the vitality would not be lessened quicker than it could be replenished, as is the case with exercise that is all muscle-building.

As muscles developed by heavy dumb-bell exercise would be valueless in endurance work, and as muscles developed by endurance movements would be valueless in performing heavy work, why not combine the two and have muscles that are strong as well as pliable and with endurance qualities and fit for all classes of work according to desire and possible need?

XIII

THERE is very little enjoyment in merely looking on at life; there is much more thrill and excitement in being one of the players. How many times have you watched the stout, lazy-appearing fellow, trying to interest himself in an athletic event or in some demonstration of athletics going on in front of him? And how often have you observed the weak, thin individual doing the same? The fat one has amusement in his eyes, for the antics and quick movements of the youths before him interest and cheer him. The thin one will have a different expression. His will be one of admiration and envy combined; his longing to duplicate the movements of the performers before him is much keener than that of his stout friend. But both of them would be much better off by participating in some form of activity than by idly sitting and watching, either eagerly or amusedly. The longer the fat man sits the lazier and stouter he becomes, and the longer the thin man waits the weaker he becomes.

Inactivity is a forerunner and a cause of decay. If you strapped your arm to your side for thirty days you would be astounded at the difference in size between the arm that was strapped and the free arm. I daresay the strapped arm would lose several inches in girth, and any bit of muscle and strength that it had possessed would be practically gone at the expiration of that time. As long as physical activity is essential, I cannot understand how anyone would purposely neglect his body and allow it to accumulate fatty tissue or, should he not be inclined to take on weight, become thinner and weaker and more sickly. What enjoyment can such types of youths and men really get out of life?

There is more to life than working, eating and sleeping. Life should be considered a privilege, and not an obligation. To the one who is overburdened with weight and whose internal organs are sluggish, it is an effort to move about; consequently he rests considerably more than does the thin, fidgety, nervous individual. The stout man puffs from the least exertion, and were he to run the short distance of one hundred feet he might experience heart pains, not to mention breathlessness and fatigue. It is an effort for him to climb stairs. If he but realized, he would feel vastly different if he adopted physical culture, he would have much more vitality, and he would have much less desire to sit around and do little or nothing. He most certainly would take more pleasure in his experiences than from any artificial thrills that money can buy. Outside of being able to float on the water, the fat man is practically helpless when it comes to saving his own life. He cannot run, he cannot jump, he cannot climb; and, in addition, when ordinary physical exertion is required he needs help.

The thin man possesses more irritability of muscle than the stout one and, naturally, is more inclined towards activity. Even though his body may be weak, his mind is willing. However, the thin man is more inclined to follow endurance work; and, therefore, as long as endurance movements are natural with him he should stick to that until he has obtained the vitality, energy and health that will give him the ambition to adopt heavier training methods.

The stout man, of course, must first of all exercise to reduce the superfluous flesh covering his muscles, for with too much fatty tissue he cannot expect ever to have any amount of endurance. His ambitions may not be as high as those of the thin, sickly man who has awakened to the value of health and strength in all their phases; but every stout man surely longs to be rid of some of his fat with as much longing as his sluggish desires permit. If formerly he had possessed sufficient ambition and energy he never would have become fat; he never would have allowed the belt to become gradually tighter around his waist. But physical laziness creeps upon one very insidiously.

A few minutes of bending and twisting movements soon will reduce his waistline, much more rapidly than he may imagine; and as he goes further into physical culture methods he will find himself gradually becoming more interested in strength work than in endurance work. This progression is natural, because the less flesh one has on one's bones (within reason) the more rapid of movement one becomes, while fat people are slow-moving individuals, and are apt to take to slow motion (strength) exercise. After reducing his waist the fat man should interest himself in strengthbuilding exercise until he has enough strength and development to be able to handle his body with ease. At that time it will be quite natural for him to interest himself in endurance movements. Although a stout man may be possessed of much patience, he would find himself becoming very impatient if he were compelled to undergo endurance work at first. Of course, there are exceptions to this general tendency. I am basing my statement upon personal observations and experience with thousands of individuals during my lifetime of teaching.

In these ways the thin man and the stout man can eventually obtain the muscular activity both in strength and endurance to be fully capable of protecting themselves in emergencies.

If you are fairly well developed and athletically inclined, perhaps what I am writing may not especially interest you; but let it be a warning to you always to keep in condition. But if by chance you are a reader to whom these words "hit home," why not now, before you lay this book aside, resolve to take up physical culture in all its branches?

The size and shape of the muscles often indicate their quality, though there are exceptions to this. I believe that muscles which are trained down to a fine point never will possess the endurance qualities of muscles that are covered by a slight fatty tissue. In the first place, a muscle that is used excessively is continually tearing down tissue; and if the muscle consists of nothing but muscle fibre continual movement will be forced action, drawing heavily upon the nervous energy. If there is a little fatty tissue covering the muscle, this tissue will be burned up first before the muscle is forced to act solely by nervous energy.

I do not mean that an arm, for example, necessarily must be fat in appearance in order to possess endurance qualities, for anyone who has seen photographs of George Hackenschmidt, the former world's champion wrestler, knows what huge, knotty muscles this famous athlete possessed; and yet he had remarkable endurance powers. His muscles, however, were not cordy or trained down to the degree of those of Eugen Sandow. Sandow undoubtedly possessed the most symmetrically developed body and the finest muscle contour of any athlete, either in this or recent past generations. Yet it is not on record that Sandow accomplished anything in the way of endurance; his muscles were remarkable for immediate action and lifting of enormous weights. But I doubt very much if Sandow in his heyday possessed half the endurance of most of our present day boxers, runners, or swimmers.

Sandow must have performed an untold amount of work and exerted tremendous effort in order to attain the physical perfection he possessed; but he probably never did any endurance movements to any appreciable extent. Hackenschmidt, on the other hand, brought heavy dumbbell exercise into his training program; but he also was a wrestler and often wrestled for hours at a time, and it was these long periods of wrestling that gave him the huge and powerful muscles, wind and endurance that he possessed.

I have seen many marvelously developed athletes whose muscles stood out in huge knobs all over their bodies and who were very pleasing to look at, but I could tell at a glance that their muscles were incapable of performing endurance work.

It may be of interest to relate a personal experience, showing how the muscles undergo a change from time to time. About ten years ago my upper arm measured relaxed thirteen and a half inches, and when flexed sixteen and a half inches. This difference of three inches was brought on by the contractile power I had in my biceps and triceps. I had developed my arms by progressive exercising, such as I am teaching today to my students who are desirous of becoming strong and muscular. Upon becoming interested in endurance work I found, after adding endurance movements to my daily exercising period and combining them with my muscleand strength-building exercise, that after a few years my upper arm still remained the same when flexed, sixteen and a half inches, but when relaxed it measured fourteen and a half inches, showing a gain of one inch in tissue and losing one inch in contractile expansion or flexion. The contour of the muscle remained practically the same when flexed, but when relaxed my arms now appeared considerably thicker than they did in the years before I became interested in endurance movements.

Perhaps you may become somewhat discouraged by my experience and the fact that, though I have continued to exercise for so many years, my arm has remained the same in size. So let me call your attention to the fact that I am no longer a "kid," and my desires to become as large as possible are over. Now I am exercising daily merely to keep in condition and to retain the development that I built up through my previous progressive efforts. I no longer perform progressive work to any marked degree, so far as muscle-building and strength exercises are concerned; for I am firm in my belief that, as I have elsewhere related, to continue progressive work year after year as one nears middle life is unwise and may bring on disastrous results. When once you have developed your body, a little light activity will keep it in shape.

The only thing you can progress in, then, is endurance; and endurance movements, if not carried too far, will prove of great benefit not only to the muscular system but to your internal organs as well. When you are doing anything calling for endurance your heart and other organs will tell you when to stop, and the only time you should continue endurance movements beyond this point is when you are in competition and some destination or goal compels you to continue. But unless you are thoroughly prepared to withstand such attacks upon your body, you will find that disastrous results will follow.

For example, it would be foolhardy for you to enter a marathon race if you never have run more than a mile or two before. It would be equally foolhardy for you to attempt to swim for a mile if the farthest distance you have heretofore made was half a mile. A boxer never would attempt to fight twenty rounds if on numerous occasions during his preparatory training for the contest he had not been able to box much more than twenty rounds.

Only the other day I entered a pool for a swim. I decided that I would swim a mile. Now many times before I had made this distance, but on this particular day the air was chilly, my muscles were cold, and my stomach was empty, and the thought of the next meal was a pleasant one. However, I dived into the water with full intentions of making the distance, fifty-three laps to the mile. Lap after lap I crawled through the water, but at about the thirtyfifth lap I felt as though I had had enough. Some inward physical warning told me not to continue. I could feel the first dull pull at my heart—that feeling that is experienced by anyone performing endurance work. Immediately I came out of the water. I believe that had I gone the other eighteen laps and completed the mile swim I might have overtaxed my heart, perhaps not dangerously but enough temporarily to interfere with its rhythmic beat and action; and every physician will tell you that continued forced muscular exertion, stimulating heart action and producing strain, eventually will cause dilatation and perhaps permanent enlargement or valvular leakage.

So, if ever you are performing exercises of endurance you should always be guided by the feeling of your organs, just as you are guided by the feeling in your stomach when it is calling for food, or the dryness of your mouth when you crave water. If you go against the laws of nature you will bring trouble upon yourself. Therefore, in all endurance exercises be sure to progress in moderation.

XIV

As SEVERAL times previously I have stated, what are exercises of endurance for one may be muscle-building work for another. Hence, experimenting must or should be done by the individual himself, to determine in what class certain exercises belong, so far as he is concerned individually. As endurance work places a heavy demand upon the lungs, and also as most forms of leg work tire the respiratory organs quicker than any other type of movements, it is necessary that special attention should be applied to all leg exercises.

The common deep knee bending exercise consists of squatting down until practically sitting on the heels and then rising again until the legs are straight. This really is a movement of endurance, for, with a little practice, it can be done hundreds of times without stopping. In the beginning, however, to one who never before has fully bent his knees ten times, it quickly will cause fatigue; but rapid progress can be made in this exercise so that after a few months one, two or three hundred repetitions can be made before the student becomes winded or the muscles tired. This indicates the rapidity with which endurance will follow the determination and use of proper methods to acquire it.

After you can perform one hundred and fifty or two hundred deep knee bends without stopping or becoming winded, you must have resistance to work against, or a barbell or someone sitting on your shoulders, to make this movement a muscle-building one. As your legs become stronger and your wind improves, the continued practice of deep knee bending or squatting with the same weight on your shoulders day after day will make this an endurance movement, for the legs will have become so muscular and strong and the wind will have become in such excellent condition that one hundred or more repetitions readily can be performed—unless the weight is increased as the legs become accustomed to the work. By the continual increasing of the weight or resistance the work becomes progressive, and naturally comes under the classification of musclebuilding exercise.

For the individual well along in years or the one with a weak heart, no progressive work should be indulged in, and the deep knee bending exercise, if done at all, should be performed very slowly, with a slight pause after each movement so as to give the heart, wind and thigh muscles a chance to recuperate. In this manner endurance movements can be performed, regardless of what the individual's organic condition may be, except, of course, serious cases under medical care; and progress can be made in added repetitions rather than in progressive resistance.

For instance, let us say that ten counts will be sufficient for the beginner who never has bent his knees in exercise. After three months he easily can perform one hundred repetitions; after six months, two hundred; and so on. Of course, such exercising would become very monotonous if no objective were in view; for this reason a limit should be drawn as to the amount of endurance work desired. If you intended to use your thighs and wind in mountain climbing, naturally it would be advantageous to you to be able to perform five hundred deep knee bends without stopping, as this would help you greatly in your proposed climb; you would find that the endurance you had acquired from the deep knee bending exercise would help you greatly in walking up steep grades, step over step. If you did not indulge in such exercise before attempting a long and laborious mountain climb you would experience fatigue before making much headway up the mountain. But if you did not contemplate performing such a pastime or any other strenuous indulgence that would be a test of your endurance powers, it would be absurd to attempt to work up to five hundred deep knee bends, for what would be the object? Without a definite objective I am sure that between one hundred and two hundred deep knee bends would give you sufficient endurance in the muscles of your thighs for all ordinary demands of daily life or emergencies.

For the muscles below the knee, the ordinary rising on the toes is an exercise that can be continued for a great number of counts. If this work is to be made progressive, you must work against a strong resistance such as by elastic or spring exerciser, or hold a bar-bell, or a heavy weight at your side while performing this movement. But as the calves are used continually in every-day walking, they are naturally somewhat hardened against exercise so that they cannot be enlarged easily, and yet they are capable of great endurance. Even the average individual, unaccustomed to any form of physical activity, has muscles of the calves capable of propelling the body in walking for great distances. The size of the calves does not need to be given any consideration in respect to endurance. I have seen men with large muscular legs who tired very quickly in walking, and others whose legs had absolutely no muscular shape whatever who were capable of walking mile after mile without giving their legs a thought.

As for preparing the muscles of the calves for endurance, I think that the best form of exercise would be heel-and-toe walking. In beginning this heel-and-toe walking you will find that the muscles of the shin play a more important part than do the muscles of the calves, as they will tire more quickly. Of course, the heel-and-toe walk is really muscle-building work for the beginner, but for the experienced walker it becomes an endurance exercise. It will be logical exercise, then, for strengthening the muscles of the shin in order to give the region below the knee greater endurance.

If you sit down in a chair and lift your feet off the floor, point your toes downward and then bring them upward toward the knee as far as they will go, you will find a strain placed upon the muscles on the outside of each shin. By bending your ankles upward and downward in this manner you exercise these muscles. Roller skating and ice skating tire these muscles of the shin very quickly, as you have found out for yourself if you do any skating.

If while sitting in a chair with your feet off the floor you are capable of raising and lowering your toes for a few hundred repetitions, you will give these muscles excellent work which will help you greatly in your endurance work performed with the legs. Deep knee bending, of course, brings into play these muscles to an appreciable extent. And while it is true that you are exercising chiefly the muscles of the thigh in performing the deep knee bend, nevertheless as the other muscles are brought into play the exercise is classified under group work; and muscles exercised in groups always have more power and coordination than muscles developed individually.

The hips also come into action in practically all forms of leg work, and strong hips are to be desired. The finest exercise for the hips that I know of is to walk rapidly through the water when it is about knee deep. By plunging forward, taking as long steps as possible, you will find that you quickly will become fatigued in the hip region. Also, walk backward in the water as rapidly as possible.

There are many who cannot do this exercise except when in bathing and many have no bathing facilities. These must indulge in other forms of hip movements. I suggest reclining work; that is, exercises performed while lying on the back, abdomen, and either side, and raising the legs upward from these positions. These exercises give direct exercise to the hip muscles.

Walking up a step grade or up flights of stairs also is an excellent movement for the hips, but such work borders on muscle-building exercise unless, through practice, you are able to walk up twenty or thirty flights of stairs without experiencing fatigue, or if you are able to walk up a steep grade for a quarter of a mile or more without becoming breathless, you can secure excellent endurance work for the hips by such exercise.

The arms always have interested me. I have enj oyed beholding massive, knotty muscles, and it is my opinion and belief that the arms never can become too large in size. I have seen so many strong men with splendid necks, fine chests and backs, and well developed legs, whose arms spoiled the contour of their physiques owing to the fact that they lacked proportionate size. Every time you move your arms you use your chest, shoulder and back muscles, as well as, in certain movements, the muscles covering the abdomen. Because of this, it is my opinion that special attention should be given to the arms, so long as they move practically all other parts of the upper body.

Do not misunderstand me, and think that you should neglect the shoulders, back and chest because of this statement. You should exercise the other muscles just the same, but you should give a little more thought to and put a little more effort into your upper arms. Strong arms are in demand and need many times; and their coordination with the shoulders, back and chest will prove invaluable in performing endurance work.

One of the most valuable arm exercises of which I know and which will bring into play also the abdomen, chest, shoulders and back, is rope-climbing. To be able to climb hand over hand up a rope, time and time again, is really an endurance feat. That it requires great strength is true; but as the repetitions can be performed many counts it should be classed as endurance work, just as lifting a fiftypound dumb-bell overhead three or four hundred times should be classed as an exercise of endurance. To lift a fifty-pound dumb-bell once is strength work for the beginner, and to endeavor to climb the rope seems quite a stunt to the average individual; but it is something that should be mastered, for the coordination and endurance that you will acquire from this exercise may prove invaluable in saving your own life or that of another.

The triceps muscle on the back of the arm can get sufficient work by the dipping exercise. This may be performed while lying flat on the floor and pushing up with the body rigid, or it can be performed between two chairs or parallel bars. In either case one can progress until able to perform the floor dip over one hundred counts and the dip between parallel bars over fifty counts without stopping because of fatigue.

To obtain coordination between the muscles used in ropeclimbing and those used in dipping between parallel bars, I suggest and strongly urge you to include a little horizontal bar work into your program. If you have no horizontal bar convenient, the same work can be done on the side of a fence, on a partition wall, or on any other object that you can reach from the ground. First pull yourself up until your chin looks over the bar, fence, or other support, then pull upward a little higher until you are able to place one elbow over the bar or fence. Then quickly place the other elbow over, and finally pull up until both arms are straight and you are resting entirely on your hands with the bar or fence rail at your hips. In other words, you should be able to climb over a fence or any object that is in your way in one continuous motion. This movement will give you coordination between your biceps and triceps and would be of great value should the occasion ever arise for you to save yourself by climbing. Actual rowing is an excellent exercise, also, for developing the biceps and triceps and coordination between these muscles.

By the above it will be understood that I advocate outdoor exercises as well as indoor exercises for the obtaining of endurance. I know from my training experience that unless you actually perform open-air sports or pastimes calling for endurance you never will become proficient in them. You can exercise faithfully in your bedroom, perform the deep knee bending movement, many times daily, do calf and shin work and the hip work until the muscles ache, and yet if you were put to the test of running up-hill you would find your respiratory organs sadly lacking in endurance. For satisfactory results you should combine indoor exercises with actual endurance work out of doors.

The same principle can be illustrated by swimming movements. After learning the motions of the crawl stroke, while you are lying in your bed or on a cot you can go through every motion with your arms, shoulders and even to the fluttering of your feet. Yet if you had had no actual experience in swimming you would lose the coordination learned in land swimming as soon as you hit the water. Of course, the knowledge of the movement would go a long way towards helping you to master actual swimming in a shorter time than without this knowledge.

But even though you were able to swim and stayed out of the water for a year or more and simply performed the movements of swimming, you would not be able to swim such distances from such practice as you would if you did actual swimming daily. It is like learning boxing in the privacy of your own room. It reads good on paper, and as you shadow-box you knock out every imaginative opponent with whom you are boxing; but even with such knowledge, and experience, were you to put on the gloves with a fairly experienced boxer you would be found wanting.

The only thing that you actually can do in the privacy of your own bedroom is to build up your body. You cannot learn to excel in any sport and you cannot obtain endurance indoors. Such quality of movement must be done in actual practice.

Competition is the greatest means of obtaining this practice and you would do well to indulge in as many forms of competitive exercise as possible. Let us suppose that you are a fairly good swimmer and that you can swim a quarter of a mile before experiencing fatigue. If you had someone who could swim a little better than you to swim with you for the same distance it would force you to make better time in the water. Perhaps the first time you might experience great discomfort at the completion of the quartermile swim; but after a while it would become easy, and a half-mile swim would interest you more than ever before.

Rarely does anyone extend himself to his limit of speed or endurance without competition or self-preservation in view. If you should be in the habit of starting out alone to take cross-country runs, endeavoring to see how quickly you can make certain distances at a rather brisk trot, you would be surprised at the much better time in which you would make similar distances if someone were racing or even running with you. And you might smash all records if you were running for your life.

It can be appreciated, then, that incentive plays an important part when it comes to extending ourselves. Just as it is quite difficult for an individual living alone to exercise day after day to build up his body, so it is difficult for an individual to adhere steadily to efforts to obtain or increase his endurance powers all by himself. Where two or more people exercise together, each one taking turns at performing movements and each one trying to outdo the other, rapid progress can be made in body building, just as track records are broken in competition which never would be broken if the runner or hurdler, or whatever he may be, were performing the work alone.

It is not the purpose of this book to give you a great variety of exercises for body-building or movements that you should follow to obtain endurance. I have herein mentioned but a few of the best movements or exercises, merely as suggestions; but experience will teach you, through the practice you will undergo with your exercising, the best movements or series of movements for your case.

In another book, Muscle Building, I have gone more fully into anatomical conditions and specific exercises.

I repeat that the main object of these pages on endurance is to awaken you fully to a realization of the value of the possession of coordination, strength and endurance sufficient to save your own life—or that of another, possibly someone more dear to you than your own life. However, I hope you will never be put to the test. Anyway, I hope the suggestions and advice contained in these pages will arouse enough enthusiasm within you to make your sports and pastimes more enjoyable.

XV

IT IS almost unbelievable what the human body can endure. To the average person it seems impossible that a man can outrun a horse; and yet it has been done. But the runner who can accomplish this probably does not think any more of it than does the average office worker of going out on his day of recreation and playing a game of baseball or indulging in some other pastime, to give his inactive muscles the activity for which they are craving.

My friend, Ottley Coulter, knowing that I contemplated writing a book of this nature, was kind enough to supply me with a few records of endurance feats, which he thought might interest my readers. I am giving them to you just as I received them. Some seem almost incredible—but there are the records! I sincerely hope that none of you will be foolish enough to attempt to beat them, for, as I told you previously in this book, my main object in offering it to you was to help you attain that degree of strength and endurance as would enable you to save your own life. Aspiring to dance, run, swim, or what not, longer than anyone else is, in my opinion, folly. All you should strive for in the physical line is robust health, vitality and a well-proportioned body. To try to become a muscular monstrosity and to strive for laurels that will prove an organic and physical impossibility may probably mean creating a mental obsession that will be just as much of a drain upon your system and life as that obsession caused by breaking the Tenth Commandment in hectic lustful cravings.

Max Danthage of Vienna, Austria, performed the deep knee-bend 6,000 times in four consecutive hours, on June 4, 1899.

Max Danthage on April 19, 1899, pressed with two hands, 74.9 pounds 845 times and followed this with 1,505 knee-bends.

Georg Ernst, on March 27, 1899, at Vienna, pressed 84.2 pounds 720 times in half an hour, and in the following hour performed 1,450 knee-bends.

4-pound dumb-bell put up, one hand, 6,000 times in 59 minutes and 53 seconds at Lynn, Mass., on June 22, 1885, by Ed. C. Stickney.

10-pound dumb-bell put up, one hand, 8,431 times in 4 hours and 34 minutes at New York, December 13, 1870, by H. Pennock.

12-pound dumb-bell put up 14,000 times with one hand by A. Corcoran at Chicago, on October 4, 1873.

25-pound dumb-bell put up 450 times by G. W. Roche, San Francisco, Calif., November 25, 1875.

162½-pound dumb-bell, raised with one hand from floor to shoulder and then pushed to arms' length above the shoulder 36 times by Louis Cyr at Chicago, May 7, 1896. C. O. Breed lifted with one hand, from the floor, a barrel of flour weighing with fixtures, 219½ pounds, 240 times in ten minutes at Lynn, Mass., on December 13, 1884.

110-pound dumb-bell put up with one hand from the shoulder, 27 times by William Conture, weighing 149 pounds, at Bath, Me., on February 11, 1892.

Henry Saltiel put up a 71¾-pound dumb-bell 118 times, changing hands each time, Newark, N. J., June 12, 1897.

Anthony McKinley at Philadelphia, on November 28, 1895, put up a 10-pound, 1½-ounce dumb-bell 10,000 times in 2 hours, 13 minutes and 20 seconds, averaging over 75 times per minute.

Frank Delmont roller-skated 50 miles in 2 hours, 47 minutes and 45 seconds, at Buenos Ayres, S. A., on October 22, 1893.

222.7 pounds pressed on feet 241 times by Anton Endres on April 8, 1896.

Swimming

Captain Webb swam from Dover, England, to Calais, France, a distance of 35 miles, in 21 hours and 45 minutes on August 24-25, 1875.

Captain Webb swam 74 miles in 84 hours, restricted to 14 hours per day in Lambeth Baths, England, starting May 19, 1879.

T. W. Burgess swam the English Channel, Dover to Cape Grisnez, September 6-7, 1911, in 22 hours and 35 minutes.

Captain Alfred Brown swam through the Panama Canal, 48 miles, at the opening in 1914; also from the Battery, New York, to Sandy Hook, in 13 hours and 38 minutes on August 28, 1913.

10 miles, 2 hours, 30 minutes and 49 seconds—L. B. Goodwin, St. Louis, Mo., September 5, 1910.

20 miles, Dover to Ramsgate, England, 6 hours and 35 minutes—Jabez Wolfe, July 6, 1906.

34½ miles, 12 hours, 44 minutes and 28 seconds, July 10, 1910, by Charles Durborow.

23 miles, 7 hours and 1 minute—Miss Eileen Lee, London, England, June, 1916.

23 miles, 8 hours and 11 minutes—Miss Annette Kellerman of Australia, at Vienna, Austria, June 12, 1906.

36¼ miles, 10 hours and 17 minutes—Miss Eileen Lee, London, England, Thames River, August 18, 1916.

35 miles, 11 hours and 35 minutes—Miss Ida Elionsky, New York, September 24, 1916.

N. B. COYKENDALL In June, 1918, swam from Milford, Pa., to Delaware Water Gap, Pa., in Delaware River, 39 miles, in 6 hours and 22 minutes, at a flood or freshet swim (meaning high rivers after a rainfall).

In September, 1919, pulled 27 people   in 2-ton motorboat one mile with hands and feet shackled in regulation handcuffs, at Silver Lake, Fairmont, Minn.

In July, 1924, swam one mile roped to a 110-foot, 1inch rope. The police and two navy captains declared him to be absolutely helpless at the time.

About same time as above, swam 150 feet standing on his head; time, 1 minute and 45 seconds.

HENRY ELIONSKY swam continuously for over 60 miles. He started from 189th Street and Hudson River and swam to Swinburne Island in the Lower Bay and then from there to Fort Lee, N. J., and from there to Woolworth Building. The judges of the swim judged the distance or mileage to be over 60 miles. This was in August, 1914.

Swam from the Battery to Swinburne Island and returned to the Battery, a distance of over 25 miles, with hands and feet shackled. Time, 11 hours and 30 minutes.

In November, 1915, swam from Brooklyn Bridge to Bay Ridge, with hands and feet shackled and towing 7 men in a sea dory. The distance was 7 miles, and the time, 3 hours and 40 minutes.

Swam from the Battery to Fort Wadsworth in the Narrows with a 200-pound man tied on his back. Distance of 10 miles, and time, 4 hours and 50 minutes.

Swam Hell Gate bound in a straightjacket with feet tied with 15 feet of iron chain. Distance, 5 miles; time, 2 hours and 40 minutes.

Swam Hell Gate with hands and feet shackled and two men bound on back in November, 1915.

Swam from Bay Ridge to the Battery tied in a chair. He made it in 3 hours and 20 minutes.

In October, 1913, swam from Battery to within a quarter of a mile of Coney Island in 5 hours and 30 minutes. The distance was 14 miles.

At Palm Beach, Fla., hauled a sea dory containing 9 men and carried two more on his back, with his hands and feet shackled, five miles, through a heavy sea, in 2 hours and 50 minutes.

Running

15 miles, 1 hour, 20 minutes and 43.5 seconds—F. Applegarth, Stamford Bridge, London, England, July 21, 1902.

20 miles, 1 hour, 51 minutes and 54 seconds—G. Crossland, Stamford Bridge, England, September 22, 1894.

25 miles, 2 hours, 18 minutes and 57 3-5 seconds— Hank Zuna, Boston, April 19, 1921.

26 miles, 385 yards; 2 hours, 32 minutes and 35 seconds—Hannes Holehmainen, Antwerp, August 22, 1920.

30 miles, 3 hours, 17 minutes and 36 1/5 seconds—J. A. Squires, England, May 2, 1885.

45 miles, 5 hours, 32 minutes and 2 seconds—E. W. Lloyd, Stamford Bridge, England, on May 12, 1913.

50 miles, 6 hours, 13 minutes and 58 seconds—E. W. Lloyd, Stamford Bridge, England, on May 12, 1913.

100 miles, 17 hours, 36 minutes and 14 seconds—J. Saunders, New York, February 22, 1882.

100 miles, 13 hours, 26 minutes and 30 seconds— Charles Rowell, New York, February 27,1882.

200 miles, 35 hours, 9 minutes and 28 seconds— Charles Rowell, New York, October 24, 1882.

300 miles, 58 hours, 17 minutes and 6 seconds— Charles Rowell, New York, February 28, to March 2, 1882.

400 miles, 84 hours, 31 minutes and 18 seconds— James Alberts, New York, February 9,1888.

500 miles, 109 hours, 18 minutes and 20 seconds—P. Fitzgerald, New York, on week of May 2 and 3, 1888.

In a 142-hour go-as-you-please running race distances are: George Littlewood, England, 623 miles; James Alberts, United States, 621; P. Fitzgerald, 610; Charles Rowell, 602; George Noremac, 566; Frank Hart, 565; E. P. Weston, 550; H. O. Messier, 526; Peter Hegelman, 526 miles.

Walking

100 miles, 18 hours, 4 minutes and 10 1/5 seconds—T. E. Hammond, London, England, on September 12,1908.

97 miles, walked in one day by James H. Hocking, New York, Times Square to Philadelphia City Hall.

67 miles without a rest, by James H. Hocking, June 5, 1919.

600 miles, New York to Cleveland, May 30 to June 10, 1919, by James H. Hocking.

Dan O'Leary walked 100 miles in 23 hours and 54 minutes on his 79th birthday.

Dan O'Leary walked 503 miles in a 6-day race in Chicago in 1875.

Edward P. Weston, age 70, New York to San Francisco, 3,895 miles in 105 days.

Edward P. Weston, age 75, New York to Minneapolis, 1,546 miles, June 2 to August 2, 1913.

John Ennis walked from Coney Island surf to the surf in San Francisco, 4,000 miles in 80 days and 5 hours.

Mrs. David Beach walked from New York to Chicago in 42½ walking days.

Skating

25 miles, 1 hour, 31 minutes and 29 seconds—J. F. Donohue, Stamford, Conn., on January 26, 1893.

50 miles, 3 hours, 15 minutes and 59 2/5 seconds—J. F. Donohue, Stamford, Conn., on January 26, 1893.

80 miles, 5 hours, 41 minutes and 55 seconds—J. F. Donohue, Stamford, Conn., on January 26, 1893.

100 miles, 7 hours, 11 minutes, 38 1/5 seconds—J. F. Donohue, Stamford, Conn., on January 26, 1893.

Roller Skating

15 miles, 49 minutes and 15 seconds—William Blackburn, Toledo, O., 1910.

24 hours, 279 miles, 319 yards—Jesse Carey, Paris, December 25, 1910.

281 8/14 miles—Robert Wheeler, Denver, Colo., February, 1917.

Bicycle Riding

72 hours, 1,163.2 miles at Paris, by Charles W. Miller.

100 miles, 2 hours, 50 minutes and 17 2/5 seconds, by F. C. Armstrong, August 16, 1898, at London.

24 hours, 452 miles, 1,715 yards, Louis Grimm, Cleveland, O., August 25, 1895.

Rowing

50 miles, 8 hours and 55 minutes, single sculls, C. A. Barnard, near Chicago, on May 12, 1877.

91 miles, 11 hours, 29 minutes and 3 seconds, single scull, John Williams, August 13, 1832.

50½-pound dumb-bell lifted from floor, right hand only, 7,600 times, by Charles Breed, Lynn, Mass., December 2, 1882, in 1 hour and 30 minutes.

50-pound dumb-bell put up, over head, 94 times with one hand by A. A. Hylton, San Francisco, Calif., May 19, 1885.

Captain Webb swam for 74 hours with only 4 minutes rest at Scaraborough, England, August 9-12, 1880.

John P. Theis played a piano without stop for 27 hours and 19 seconds at Philadelphia on July 5, 1893.

C. A. Harriman at Truckee, Calif., on April 6-7, 1883, walked 121 miles and 385 yards without a rest.

Peter Crossland at Manchester, England, walked 120 miles and 1,560 yards on September 11-12, 1876, without a rest.

2,280 miles in 912 hours, consecutive, by William Gale, concluding at Bradford, England, May 14, 1879.

Chinning 78 times, Anton Lewis, Brockton, Mass., April, 1913.

Skipping the rope 11,810 times, J. M. Barnett, Carlisle, N. S. W., on February 5, 1913.

Martin Dobrilla swung a pair of 3-pound, 4-ounce Indian clubs 144 hours at Cobar, N. S. W., Australia. Harry J. Lawson did the same for 134 hours at Bundaberg, Australia, on March, 1913.

www.ingramcontent.com/pod-product-compliance
Lightning Source LLC
Chambersburg PA
CBHW070138290526
45789CB00002B/531